Advanced Technologies and Societal Change

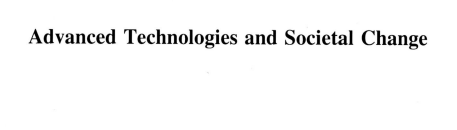

For further volumes:
http://www.springer.com/series/10038

Eckehard Fozzy Moritz

Editor

Assistive Technologies for the Interaction of the Elderly

The Development of a Communication Device for the Elderly with Complementing Illustrations and Examples

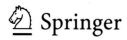 Springer

Editor
Eckehard Fozzy Moritz
Innovationsmanufaktur GmbH
Munich
Germany

ISSN 2191-6853   ISSN 2191-6861   (electronic)
ISBN 978-3-319-00677-2   ISBN 978-3-319-00678-9   (eBook)
DOI 10.1007/978-3-319-00678-9
Springer Cham Heidelberg New York Dordrecht London

Library of Congress Control Number: 2014935226

Printed on acid-free paper

Springer is part of Springer Science+Business Media (www.springer.com)

Foreword

Welcome to this book. It is a special book in many regards, not only in the way we tackled the project described, but also in the way the book itself is set up: We tried many, and partially new, ways to make it as interesting and valuable to you as possible. See for yourself, below, or on any of the pages that follow.

First of all: Whom did we address in this book? We are convinced that it will be useful for those who.

- Work in complex technological projects, especially those in which meeting the interests, motivations, and predispositions of users plays a big role.
- Address innovations for the elderly in the wake of the demographic change.
- Organize projects with partners from many backgrounds, countries, and institutions.
- Look for an example of the work on and the result of a Holistic Innovation project.

Still, the reader may think that books on technological projects are often for the most part irrelevant and hence rather boring except for those who worked on the project, and they (should) know what they did. The same goes for edited books written by many authors: While a few ideas and articles will be stimulating, others usually are not—neither in style nor in content. What you hold in your hand is a book on a technological project written by many authors. What did we do to nevertheless make it interesting for you to read?

- First of all, the book is structured according to the process of Holistic Innovation introduced in Process: How We Structured an Innovation Project Towards Maximum Use Value which should increase its dramaturgic value and might be interesting in its own right.
- Next, the authors started writing the book with a lot of common thoughts and convictions. We not only adhered to one TargetVision in the project, but we also jointly collected and organized what we think is valuable enough to be communicated to the world. We also added a few topics that did not play a big role in this project but may be of big importance in similar projects with a slightly different focus; especially how to realize "joy of use" and how to adhere to "movement motivation." We also cross-checked the chapters and had internal reviews aiding consistency and quality.

- Finally, we put (almost) all chapters into the same structure, offering an executive summary and the main results first, then describing the work in more detail, and eventually, wherever interesting or the authors felt it was needed, adding a scientific excursion.

So there you go. Process: How We Structured an Innovation Project Towards Maximum Use Value offers an overview over the process and the result of each step as well as the project itself and hence should be a must-read, possibly save the scientific excursion. The same goes for Recommendations: What We Suggest, in which we compiled everything we learned in this project so that others will be able to share the success factors and avoid the mistakes we made. For those interested in the results of the project only: These are summarized in Product: What We Generated in this Project. For any other chapter we invite you to read the headline and executive summary and decide for yourself whether the contents seem interesting or relevant to you. Certainly, the intensive work we did to understand and collaborate with the elderly is worth reading, as are many practical elements in the realization of what we did.

We hope that this book will be stimulating to you. If it is, let us know. If it is not, let us know as well and suggest how we could improve our publications in the future. Anyway, have fun reading it!

Finally, special thanks go to the authors and the publisher of this book on the one hand, and on the other hand to the sponsors and project agencies that helped us throughout the project and pushed us toward doing a good job. I personally am most deeply grateful to Steffi Erdt and Esther Zierer who had the painstaking work of putting everything together, pushing the authors (including myself), ensuring the quality of the work, and still kept my mood and motivation up. I also must not forget Martin Strehler who had the project idea, Katja Popp who set up this project and started it, and Javier Gámez Payá who continued on as project leader and kept the whole team in Spain, Italy, Austria, and Germany in line with Spanish style and charm.

Munich, March 2014   Eckehard Fozzy Moritz

Preface: A Designed Dialogue—the Editor and the Users

Dear Reader,

Yes, it is nice to have the Head of an AAL funding unit, a science minister or even Barack Obama write a preface; giving a book, and in our case also the related project, a high standing. But let us face it: neither of them would really have much of knowledge nor much of heart and empathy regarding the contents. How could they possibly?

Thus, when I was pondering who should write such a preface I soon realized who would be the perfect authors, combining intimate knowledge with heart and empathy regarding the contents of this book: It is the users, the very active, interested and supportive group of elderly people who helped us make the SI-Screen/Elisa project such a success. They accompanied our innovation from the very start: From telling us what social interaction means to them to testing the third prototype in their own homes.

The theory infusing this collaboration and examples of its impact are addressed in various chapters of this book, but the actual voice of the elderly is hardly heard. So in what follows I "design" a short dialog as, or one may say instead of, a preface, summarizing some typical questions we asked and throwing in original answers of our valued collaborators. With this I like to devote the whole book to those whom we addressed in our project, and who helped us so much throughout the work on it. Thank you so much, dear users in Spain, and dear users in Germany.

"You told us you don't use communication technologies much. Why is that so?"

"I'm afraid to touch something because my children work with computers and they tell me off if I change the configuration of something."

"And it all changes from one day to the next; and you need the whole morning to re-learn everything."

"But you appear to like communication? Why don't you like the computer for that?"

"It's not the same, it's cold."

"Many people are excluded by the Internet! It always says if you want to know more, please look it up on the Internet!"

"The non-verbal communication is very important. Technology cannot replace that."

"For me, it is idiotic when people walk and at the same time talk on their mobile phones."

"You said you did use communication technologies at times. Do you remember any positive experiences?"

"When my grandchildren stayed in Australia, I had more contact to them via Skype than I have today."

"Yes, Skype is fantastic. But I do not know how to install it."

"Before everybody had the possibility [to connect to the Internet], contacts to former colleagues were rare, because everybody was so busy. Maybe you would have called every second week, now you have contact every second day."

"Ten years ago, I hated e-mail accounts, now I hate people who don't have an e-mail account! It is the same with computers and the Internet."

"And are there things you are really afraid of?"

"What I will not do is Facebook. You never know what happens with the data."

"And I do not know what we want to do with the entire information flood."

"I cannot establish contacts via the Internet—that is something for younger people."

"I am still afraid of the computer, because I think: It will win against me!"

"Maybe you can also tell us about some specific experiences?"

"The worst ever was to reach the telephone hotline of the train."

"PCs are frustrating—I do not find what I want, I do not see properly—and nobody has the patience to explain it to me."

"PCs are dangerous—you can make a lot of mistakes and you will see them on the telephone bill."

"Since the cable broke I do not have access to the Internet anymore."

"Well, we have the idea to develop a social interaction device entirely tailored to your needs, interests, and wishes. What do you think about this, what would you like about it?"

"I would love to try it and to have the possibility to join [the Internet]."

"I have a friend who helps me with smaller problems with the computer via Team Viewer. But for larger problems, it would be nice to have a hotline that you can always call. I would even pay for this."

"If I had internet, I would do that [booking flights] by myself."

"It is good to have someone in my circle of friends, who is familiar with the Internet."

"So, now you have tested our solution; even our third prototype. What do you think?"

"Before the test I was very skeptical, but then I was pleasantly surprised by the Elisa system and its possibilities!"

"It helps to find just the information I am interested in."

"You can find somebody to go for a walk or something else—it is like an Elisa community."

"Can you tell us about your most interesting experiences?"

"After three days I had learned all about the Elisa system. I think it is very good for people who don't use computers."

"At the beginning I had big problems, but then it got better and better and in the end I even had fun!"

"The way you move to other pages is really simple and the font size seems adequate."

"And your final judgment?"

"I think Elisa could be a real chance to enlarge social contacts."

"It is an opportunity to find other people with similar interests."

Munich, March 2014   Eckehard Fozzy Moritz

Contents

Contributors

Ricard Barberà-Guillem, Instituto de Biomecánica de Valencia

Stephan Biel, Tioman & Partners SL

Martin Burkhard, Universität der Bundeswehr München

Nadia Campos, Instituto de Biomecánica de Valencia

Isacco Chiaf, Helios

Marc Delling, Silpion IT-Solutions GmbH

Stefanie Erdt, Innovationsmanufaktur GmbH

Javier Gámez Payá, Innovationsmanufaktur GmbH

Steffen Ganz, Porsche Design Studio

Javier Ganzarain, Tioman & Partners SL

Jan Kliewer, Helios

Michael Koch, Universität der Bundeswehr München

Gustavo Monleón, Servicios de Teleasistencia

Eckehard Fozzy Moritz (Editor), Innovationsmanufaktur GmbH

Andrea Nutsi, Universität der Bundeswehr München

Hannes Pasqualini, Helios

Wilhelm Prasser, Data United GmbH

Martin Strehler, Innovationsmanufaktur GmbH

Fee Wiebusch, Brainware GmbH

Ute Vidal Cabello, VIOS Medien GmbH

Abbreviations

AAL	Ambient Assisted Living
Elisa	Elderly interaction and service assistant (product name)
EMS	Electronic manufacturing services
EU	European Union
G2M	Go to market
GUI	Graphical user interface
HCI	Human-computer interaction
IBV	Instituto de Biomecánica de Valencia
ICT	Information and communication technology
IOP	Innovación orientada a las personas (user-oriented innovation)
iOS	iPhone operating system
IPR	Intellectual property rights
IT	Information technology
JP	Joint programme (a EU funding program)
MVC	Model view controller
NUI	Natural user interfaces
OEM	Original equipment manufacturer
OS	Operating system
R&D	Research and development
SDK	Software development kit
SI-Screen/Elisa	Social interaction screen (project name)
SME	Small and medium enterprises
SMS	Short message service
SNS	Social network service
SSIL	Social software integration layer
T&C	Terms and conditions
TP 55	Treffpunkt 55plus (a Munich-based organization providing services for the elderly)
UI	User interface
UniBwM	Universität der Bundeswehr München
USP	Unique selling proposition
WHO	World Health Organization
WIMP	Windows, icons, menus, pointing

Process: How We Structured an Innovation Project Towards Maximum Use Value

Eckehard Fozzy Moritz, Stefanie Erdt and Javier Gámez Payá

1 Executive Summary

In this chapter, in fact in the whole book, we will aim at illustrating rationale and process of the methodology of Holistic Innovation, which is maximizing the gross value of an innovative development for its intended users from the very onset of the project. We will argue that such a project must start with an identification of a worthwhile topic area, and with an in-depth understanding of the characteristics of the user groups, and what sort of functional values they are interested in, even including interests that they are not aware of yet. It is furthermore vital to know in which environment and with what kinds of resources the innovation will need to be realized. Only on such a basis do the usual starter activities like creative concept finding and system layout make sense. The subsequent process of successive realization and optimization should be organized in intense rounds of collaboration with the user groups. Finally, even though principal market reflections should accompany the project discussions from the very start, a more concrete planning of value chains and production and distribution channels must also become an important part of the system development, so that the innovation can emerge into full beauty from an individual and social as well as an economic perspective.

2 Main Results

The main steps of the process introduced here are summarized in Fig. 1, complemented by the core results achieved in the project. This graphical representation of process rationale and results has been used at conferences and in project meetings ever since the first public presentation of Elisa at the European AAL

E. F. Moritz (✉) · S. Erdt · J. Gámez Payá
Innovationsmanufaktur GmbH, Munich, Germany
e-mail: efm@innovationsmanufaktur.com

E. F. Moritz (ed.), *Assistive Technologies for the Interaction of the Elderly*,
Advanced Technologies and Societal Change, DOI: 10.1007/978-3-319-00678-9_1,
© Springer International Publishing Switzerland 2014

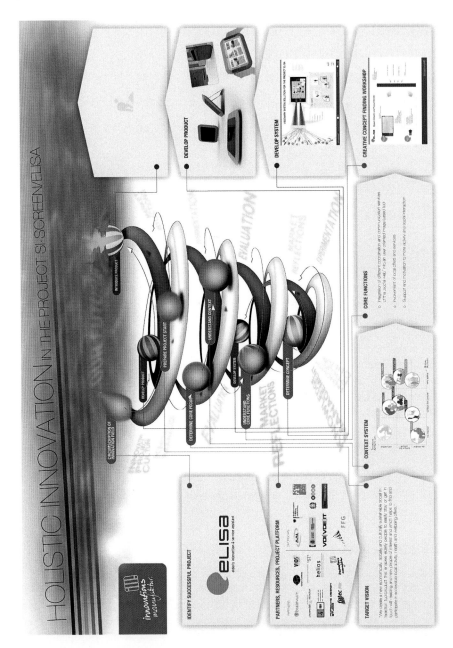

Fig. 1 Process rationale, steps and respective results of the project SI-Screen/Elisa

Forum in Lecce in September 2011. To avoid any confusion: The official name of the whole project is "Social Interaction Screen" (SI-Screen/Elisa), whereas the developed product/prototype is called "elderly interaction and service assistant" (Elisa).

Of course, as the project progressed, the graphic was continuously adjusted, so that by today the results of all steps are illustrated or at least exemplified in the respective field. Further details of the results can be found later in this chapter, and in subsequent chapters of this book.

3 Storyline

In this book, the story of the project SI-Screen/Elisa is told, the development of an innovative product and system solution that will much improve social interaction and integration of elderly people. This chapter is devoted to the process we applied, mainly its use value, but also its pitfalls.

Even though the process of Holistic Innovation had been successfully applied for more than eight years now in myriads of projects, the project SI-Screen/Elisa really constituted the first utilization of this methodology in a large scale European project. One main reason for this is that this methodology is not easy to align with traditional funding schemes: We much appreciated that we were allowed at all to conduct the project without having to define the details of the solution beforehand—which should be a matter of course but often is not, not even in projects aiming at innovation. But we soon experienced that very few project partners had any prior experience with this way of tackling innovation projects.

Among other things, this had two ramifications: During the first half of the project many project partners had quite some difficulties to adjust to the new process approach. Especially the fact that the eventual concept and system design were only realized after more than six months into the project, that they were preceded by alternating steps of embedding, focusing, and decision making, that even user involvement began well before a clear project prospective could be communicated, appeared rather disturbing to the usual working habits of many members of the team. By the second half of this project, however, all this had changed. Not only did tasks and focus become very clear, it also became obvious that the approach applied had been perfectly useful: The concept design turned out to be right to the point of user interests and likes, was embedded into a system environment in which all pieces fit together well, and still could be realized in a modular approach by the appropriate partners. Best of all, the team members themselves liked the result, and "wanted to have one", even though none of them was/is in the target group. And, as evidenced by first talks, investors and producers share the team's enthusiasm: At the time of writing, the realization of Elisa as a whole new system solution facilitating, in many cases even enabling, communication and social integration of the elderly is being planned in a very promising business setting.

How did all of that come about; and especially, what did the process leading to such a successful innovation and the corresponding work look like? In the following, we will describe more closely the work on and the results of the different process steps summarized in Fig. 1, and add some backstage stories wherever they can lead to new conceptions or other insights. A more elaborate discussion of the work done in the following steps can be found in the subsequent chapters of this book.

Circumscription of an innovation field: identify a successful project

The topic area of this innovation project was more or less given by the formulation of the call for projects published by the AAL Joint Programme: "ICT based solutions for advancement of social interaction of elderly people".

Of course, this point of entry into a project is a consequence of the current habits in much of the project sponsoring by public institutions who by the formulation of a call decide upon the main purpose and the direction of impact. In an overall view of Holistic Innovation activities to shape the future, the very core of an innovation venture may start at a much earlier stage; in a discourse about how a desirable future for the stakeholders could look like, where resources and competences are located, which boundary conditions and innovation enablers exist and hence in which fields and with what objectives concrete projects should be launched.

Most of this having been pre-determined, it was nevertheless important to define a specific objective for a project that needed to serve at least three purposes: Following the lines of our own self-understanding, it had to have maximum positive impact for the intended target group, the elderly. For the sponsors, it had to be compatible enough to other projects and their lines of action and it had to be communicable to, at the very least, politicians and potentially critical media. And lastly, it had to be well-founded enough so that the experts evaluating the proposal would find enough of their own convictions and reasoning to evaluate the project proposal positively and thus make sure that it would be granted. Dear reader, if you think this is all more or less the same, believe us it is not. However, a further discourse on this matter clearly exceeds the scope of this chapter.

What we came up with as a compromise of all of this, also taking into account our own competences and those of our core partners (with whom we had intense discussions already at this point), was the following essence of the project description: "Wellbeing and social interaction: improving the quality of life of the elderly and strengthening their social interaction with a digital social interaction tool".

Prepare project start: partners, resources, project platform

Regarding the resources, the order of magnitude in the amount of funding was more or less indicated by what is typical in such project applications. Of course, given the immense work such an application is, and the great uncertainty of whether an application will be successful or not (the success rates range from 3 to 30 % of all applications), one would try to get most income out of an application and not go for small scale projects.

There is more about resources, however, that is usually forgotten. In innovation projects in which the concrete objective and the specific work to be done is deliberately not well defined at the onset, there has to be benevolent trust among the core partners, a positive chemistry, as a basis for the ease and fun of collaboration with nonetheless (or for exactly that reason?) efficient work and productive results, and a positive image to the inside and outside world (see also Moritz and Ruth 2007). To give just some examples, there has been a long and successful collaborative working history between Innovationsmanufaktur and the partners from the Universität der Bundeswehr München, close emotional and ideological bonding with core partners in Valencia, and quickly established informal ties with the team from Porsche Design, all this complementing the core criteria of a perfect fit of project partners with respect to competence, quality, and reliability.

In terms of web-based collaboration platforms, the project experiences also deviated from what may be thought to be mainstream action. At the beginning, after quite some consultation, we chose and put lots of efforts into installing Comindwork (www.comindwork.com), which promised "a radical way to structure communication. Your teams will escape email noise, file chaos and will bring accountability to work." Nevertheless, apparently most of the team rather appreciated email noise, file chaos and less accountability, for the sake of use flexibility and not having to acquaint themselves with yet another platform. Thus mailing lists, conference calls, frequent direct meetings—also with users—and the semi-annual project meetings really were the key "collaboration" elements.

Determine core focus: TargetVision

Once the project thus got started, the next step according to the Holistic Innovation process was the definition of the TargetVision, the condensation of all aspects of stakeholder objectives and interests that will determine the basic design of the solution concept. A TargetVision usually only consists of one or two sentences, possibly including an itemization, and serves as a tool for motivation, orientation, and coordination of efforts for the whole team during the first stages of an innovation project, and as basis for "evaluating" the outcome later. In the first meeting of all project partners the TargetVision was determined as follows: "…to create an economically, socially and culturally sustainable social interaction tool/product that enables elderly people to easily stay or get in touch with existing and new people of interest and which helps to find and participate in accessible local activity, health and wellbeing offers."

Embed innovation: understand context system

Before ideation, it is vital to know as many relevant aspects as possible related to the environment in which the innovation will have to function. Examples are:

- A deep understanding of characteristics, motivations, and use scenarios of the later users (we hate the word "consumers"): In our project especially it was necessary to differentiate what exactly the term "elderly people" means; a huge group of the population that is all but homogenous with regards to ICT affinity and social interaction. Similar to the so-called Sinus Milieus (www.sinus-institut.de/en)

in that they are a mix of theoretical conception and focus group involvement, we defined eight types useful for our innovation task (see chapter "User Groups and Characteristics: How We Described the User Groups"). Among these, a few were selected as target groups for the Elisa development, and so-called "power users" in each of these groups became core sparring partners for all later development steps. Regarding Elisa itself, we defined among other things different use cases which described where and when Elisa could be used by the later customers. In addition, a poster on the "inner demon" was developed explaining how different types of people can be motivated to support their health and wellbeing.

- An up-to-date reflection of innovation enablers, trends and developments in relevant technologies, services, and activities: Using the current state of the art to realize an innovation and knowing what the future will bring in terms of predictable development will make sure that the solution to be developed will be as efficient as possible and for at least some time to come be compatible with other ongoing developments (all the more important in the blazing ICT innovation rage today). For Elisa, the rapid development in the field of tablets and the increased importance of the Web 2.0 were particularly interesting.
- A list of stakeholders and an understanding of their interests: In our project we discovered an amazing complexity of parties potentially involved in the product success. Complementing the diversity of our target group, the team itself and the sponsors, with AAL Europe and four national contact points, we found information and service providers of all sorts, representatives and interest groups of/ for the elderly, a wide array of potential business partners depending on the production and distribution scenarios, and many more. While this did not make our task easy, it nevertheless helped to make sure we could take into account as much of their needs and interests in the innovation process as possible, as soon as possible.

Core functions: understand and define what needs to be performed

To begin with, an innovative solution of any sort is in the first place not a product or a service, but a way to realize intended functions. Regardless whether they are technical, logistic or administrative, at the core of all innovation work there should be an understanding of the functions the solution is supposed to provide for the intended users. In a first round, interpreting the TargetVision on the basis of some environmental knowledge, we thus came up with the following list of functions:

- Integration of different coordination and communication services on the social web into one user-oriented image-based tool
- Involvement of local actors, offers and services
- Support for and motivation to more activity and social interaction

Realizing that this was far too much to realize in a high quality fashion in the framework of this one project, we narrowed down the user-oriented core functionalities to communication, information and inspiration, corresponding to what we felt was the core of the TargetVision.

Determine concept: creative concept finding

Truly, whereas concept finding usually means lots of creative inspiration and fun, in this project it was really hard, and not overly joyful, work. The task of "concepting" itself is not that difficult: You focus on the development of a concept that will realize the core functions, taking into account whatever is important of the context system, and you come up with a variety of more or less fitting ideas which you can group, optimize, synthesize, all on the way to an optimum solution. In this case, however, we had enthusiastic representatives of user groups expecting a lot on the one hand, and on the other experts in programming knowing exactly how few completely new functions can actually be realized. We had those thinking in great apparatuses and additional mobile devices, and those imagining a beautiful backend software. We had the ones that envisioned integrating all the health and social involvement services, and others who were dreaming of big buttons in a sturdy hardware. We had the old and the young, the creative and the boring, from altogether four different countries. This was, this is difficult. But we did not evade this difficulty; on the contrary, we plunged right into it. And when we saw what we finally came up with, as result of this entire struggle, the whole team was very proud: Yes, we really found a unique product that perfectly delivers what we were aiming for from the very beginning.

Develop system: from backend to health service integration

A successful innovation needs a good system design: While maybe not yet commonplace, this conviction is spreading more and more, and rightfully so. To appreciate what this statement means, and why Holistic Innovation puts so much emphasis on system design, let us just point out a few questions we addressed, and solved, during the realization of Elisa:

- How would the elderly learn about the product features, and initialize and update the software? For this purpose we developed a very simplified and truly intuitive user interface and extra tutorials, as well as a supportive backend, optimized in three rounds of testing by the target group. For anything more complex we enabled the elderly to choose a person of trust, who had complete administrator access and could perform all work necessary or sensible. For a more detailed description see chapter "Evaluation: How We Tested and Optimized Elisa".

- How could interesting information automatically be updated, with basic content and range preselected, and yet be trustful to the user? The software, Social Software Integration Layer, automatically unifies the profile data, activity streams (status updates) and content streams (comments, recommendations, photos) of existing social networking services (Facebook, Google+), social content sharing platforms (Flickr, Picasa), group calendars (Google Calendar) as well as website feeds (events, articles), mailing lists and personal blogs. This information is filtered according to the users' needs, and in order to guarantee trustable content, an organization checks the quality of the data. For a more detailed description see chapter "Social Software Integration: How We Integrated Different Interaction Features and Technologies".

- How can standard hardware be used and yet offer a highly appealing design and functionalities to the elderly? To solve this dilemma, we first determined which type and size of hardware would be the most desirable for the target group (it proved to be a mid-sized tablet), and put this into a housing whose very design would fit into the living environments of the elderly and could offer desired functions like a big switch with a definite on/off feel. For a more detailed description see chapter "Design: How We Attempted to Attract Users in Optics, Haptics, and Ease of Utilization".

Further steps: product development, business planning, and more

The subsequent steps of detailed product development and business planning went hand in hand with loads of inspiration, transpiration, and conspiracy; however, the process itself was more straightforward and less uniquely holistic in character than some of the previous activities. Details will be elaborated upon in the chapters "User Groups and Characteristics: How We Described the User Groups", "User Involvement: How We Integrated Users into the Innovation Process and What We Learned from It", "Design: How We Attempted to Attract Users in Optics, Haptics, and Ease of Utilization" and "Business: How We Worked to Get Elisa into the Market and Share the Benefits".

Further important process reflections

Much of the work in this complex innovation project could only be performed successfully because right from the beginning we focused on accompanying activities that were necessary to make the cooperative and at first ambiguous work crossing so many borders successful. To mention just a few examples:

- The focus on generative resources like trust, mutual understanding and appreciation, and the building of joint competence were not only important at the beginning, but throughout the project. All big project meetings were accompanied by intense social activities building a strong working team. By the way, those who claim that this may be a waste of the taxpayers' money be assured: Not doing so would be a waste of the taxpayers' money!
- Intensive user involvement was a prime factor for producing a fitting solution. In this case, we had worked with users and power groups even before concept finding, and we also tested the respective states of development in three rounds, finally even allowing the users to test the product at home. Complementing this we had regular meetings with groups of elderly in which current developments, needs, and wishes were discussed in informal evening settings.
- Switching between serious discussions and at times humorous changes of perspective was, although not yet applied systematically, a great help to ease tensions and make sure we would not lose focus and run into dead ends but keep the whole development well on track. We advise to use this great "tool" more extensively in future projects.

4 Scientific Excursion

First a word of warning to those readers who may expect a more traditional "scientific" excursion: In the complex matter of rationalizing a new way of looking at and structuring innovation, we will not embark on grounding all of this on previous studies and evidence in this book. Eckehard "Fozzy" Moritz has done so in his book (Moritz 2009), and needed almost 190 pages for this task alone. On the few pages we have here we will try to maximize the impact of the message; hence please forgive the almost complete lack of citations.

Nevertheless, any discussion of the process of innovation should, as it will here, start with a brief reflection on the nature of innovation: What is innovation? And why do we innovate at all? No, don't be afraid that we will start from scratch with the definitions given by the grandfather of innovation discourse, Josef Schumpeter. Still, being an economist (and maybe that is where the trouble started...), in all of his arguments he focused on two aspects of the nature of innovation: idea and market success (e.g. Schumpeter 1934). This led to myriads of further discussions and definitions along the same lines which only in very few cases really deviated from this focus.

Now, we would like to deviate from it in three aspects:

- Most importantly, we see one thing lacking that should, to our minds even must, be at the heart of any discourse on innovation: The functionalities that are to be provided by an innovation, the meaning, the sense that is being created, should be the pivotal starting point to man-made innovation. That notion will separate innovations that are merely a scam to empty people's pockets from innovations that contribute strongly to future developments desirable for the majority of stakeholders.
- Secondly, success for us must not be confined to market success. Rather, it should be regarded as success if the objective of an innovation is achieved to some satisfactory degree. If the main intention was to create market success, then, yes, Schumpeter's notion is right. But often the intentions are different, be it due to the nature of the task or to the fact that the stakeholder embarking on a particular innovation venture is not a typical market player. In our case, the European Union wanted more and better communication for and social integration of their elderly population, so if we achieve this task, by (also) creating new forms of social organization, we may consider ourselves successful. Of course, the European Union also wanted a product/system solution to be developed and distributed, and if this is done in a traditional market setting, this implies the need for a market success. But this is the means, not the end.
- Thirdly, the wording of and focus on "ideas" to us is misleading, implicating that the heureka effect is at the heart, even at the origin of innovation. To us, the importance of ideas in an innovation process is grossly overrated, at least in terms of workload and intellectual challenge. What you need to achieve in an innovation venture is the production of an efficient fitting product/system solution (fitting to needs, trends, motivations, technologies, interfaces, zeitgeist, and much more...)

and its realization and distribution to the intended target group. Just having an idea may boost egos at regular's tables, but will usually not mean much more...

Summarizing all of this, after a few decades of working on innovation projects we came up with the following definition (why do short things always take such a long time...) which eventually forms the basis of all Holistic Innovation considerations:

> Innovation is a Novelty with Sense and Success.

What does it mean for the process of creating an innovation if it is defined in such a way? The most important point is that this process should not start with novelty, with ideation, even though its positioning in the above sentence and myriads of books on innovation suggest otherwise. But it just does not make sense to produce ideas in quick rounds of inspirations and then look for sense and success, or just success. It is intellectually satisfying and an interesting educational practice to work on ideation, and ideas often initially appear great, especially to their producers. Often, people only become aware that an idea does not really fit after a lot of effort has been put into its realization; the ideas in question may realize a core function in a very creative fashion but may not be appreciated by people, be too expensive to produce, or be not manageable, not compatible, not in zeitgeist... oh, there are so many reasons why innovations fail.

This is why the process of Holistic Innovation suggests progressing differently:

- First, the stakeholders should be very clear on the overall objectives, the sense to be created in an innovation venture.
- Second, the innovators should try to define and understand what determines the later success of an innovation.
- Third, only on this basis does it make sense to produce novelty; which, much more than just quickly churning out ideas, means producing fitting concept and system solutions.
- Forth, many efforts have to be undertaken to make sure that the solution developed will also become available to the intended target group; only then success will be achieved.
- Fifth, with the success of the product/system solution the originally intended sense is hence created.

In the following, we will elaborate a little on these considerations and try to transfer them to practical process recommendations, thus backing up the procedure followed in our project and the storytelling of the previous subchapter. We will start with the following claim:

Innovation is THE means to influence the shaping of future into a desired direction...

... into "The Future We Want", as has been the fitting motto of the Earth Summit in Rio in June 2012.

Of course, in one project one cannot design the whole future; in fact, it can never be "designed" completely: Developments are too complex, and not at all deterministic, so all innovators can do is influence future to take a desired direction. But this they can. And this they should: Future happens anyway, and it is so much better and so much more responsible to think how it could and should look like, and act accordingly, rather than to let future developments become the haphazard mash-up result of all acts of those in power—which currently means an all-too-dominant focus on creating profits for a very select few rather than advancing the quality of life for all.

Considerations on sense

As one could guess from the above, we are all but convinced that economic benefit is the main "sense" of innovation; however wide-spread this thinking appears today. Profit is one essential objective and driving force for one important group of stakeholders in innovation ventures in a free market economy: private companies. But it is no more than that: We are convinced that the dominant role of thinking and acting according to short-term measurable economic benefits is not only grossly overrated in today's world in a way that is all but sustainable; it is also not the main nature of innovation. But what then is the sense of innovation? Or, phrased differently, why do we innovate, and why do we claim we need to create sense by doing so?

Let us put in a few rather philosophical considerations about how our future comes into being here. "Future" is being shaped as a synergetic complex result of all human activities, and is at the same time embedded in and dependent on changes in all sorts of environmental boundary conditions, emerging developments and happenstances. Most of our activities now are rather habitual, routines along the lines of activities that we have always been doing. If we maintain that behavior, the future will be quite similar to how we live today. However, innovation by its very nature impacts change. Innovations are an intentional deviation from habits and routines. Innovation is our main instrument to make the future different from the present.

On these premises one thought becomes quite obvious: If innovation is THE means of shaping the future, why are we not concerned much more by the question what we want our future to look like? Why do we not discuss "the future we want"? Should not the result of such a thinking ahead of the future be the main impetus for innovation, to make sure that with innovation we at least try to shape a desired and desirable future?

To be sure, it is naïve to think that with innovation projects one can determine future. As has been stated before, the overall of developments, influences and interrelations that conclude in our future is complex, chaotic, and not at all deterministic. So all innovators can do is influence the future to take a desired direction. But this they can. And this they should.

Summarizing all this, sense in innovation means the sum of collective wisdom projected onto plausible objectives and feasible opportunities for a future that is deemed attractive by most of its stakeholders. Admittedly, finding such a defined "sense" is not an easy task; one that requires lots of discourse and negotiations, productive fantasy, systemic visioning, and the generation of synergies. But, hey, is not that the true essence of directing our live and work? Hence we strongly pledge that we embark much more on discussing what is or should be the sense in innovation projects, and start from there, rather than only ever accelerating a wheel with little idea as to where it is rolling.

Considerations on success

Knowing the sense of innovation, the next thing we need to find out is what we have to acknowledge and to address to make sure that an innovation project will be successful, or at least to strongly increase the likelihood of success. Success in this context means that the intended sense is created and the objectives achieved.

One of the core ideas of Holistic Innovation in that regard is that we need to know the cornerstones of success well before we think about ideas, concepts, and structures: The solutions that we will be producing in an innovation project will need to function in a very complex system of interests, boundary conditions, existing solutions and stakeholders, with many resulting interfaces and interrelations. Most important of all: An innovation needs to be used; hence, before we start with designing a concept, we need to know what will motivate people to utilize our innovation. Innovations that are not used create neither sense nor profit. To be sure, in reasoning about preconditions of success, also economic rationalities play an important role. Which economic interests do stakeholders have, what do they mean by value creation, what price corridors may be acceptable, and other issues.

In the terminology of the Holistic Innovation methodology all of this is phrased as follows: In the preparation of concept generation we need to know about all potentially relevant dimensions of the innovation context system, and we need to know and understand the functions an innovative solution will need to perform. To stick to the project presented here, we need to know what technologies and enablers exist to produce innovative solutions for the elderly, how much money they might be able and willing to spend on average, what aspects of social interaction are of big importance to them and, most importantly, what would make them accept and use information technologies in their daily lives.

Considerations on novelty

Talking to some experts about innovation, we were quite often faced with the comment that by doing that much preparatory work before being allowed to be creative will greatly reduce the potential scope for creative solutions and hence be

very much counter-productive. However, with some clever planning and preparation of the creative concept finding you can really turn this perceived short-
coming into an advantage. The trick is to focus, direct and challenge the creative
mind to those aspects in which break-through solutions can make a difference, and
distract it from focusing on the few "typical" or fashionable things that immediately come to people's minds but do of course not grasp the whole of the project.

To give an example, in our project it made a lot of sense to really understand
what social interaction means for the elderly, how they may be grouped into different milieus, and what their respective interests, barriers, and motivators are: On
this basis we could then steer our creative minds to finding novel approaches to user
interface design, hardware shells, and backend functionalities rather than remaining
focused on fashionable app-design, however creative those apps may be.

As a practical excursion, best results in concept development have been
achieved by the following sequence of activities in a concept finding workshop.

1. Find the right heterogeneous mix of participants, to ensure synergies and
   deviations from typical thinking patterns.
2. Put them into a creative physical and mental environment far away from any
   relation to typical day-to-day work.
3. Make them understand the task, the context system, and the functions to be
   realized.
4. Have them experiment with functions, to get a physical and practical understanding of things and provide for more emphatic solutions.
5. Ask some core opening questions demanding creative answers in aspects in
   which solution finding merits creativity, truly shifting horizons and doing
   away with every day mental blinders.
6. Let all participants individually produce creative concepts, asking for quality,
   not quantity. Ingenuity is not democratic, the ideas of ALL need to be collected individually first and then discussed in the group.
7. Let participants present their concepts, and engage all to criticize produc-
   tively: How could we optimize this solution to make it work best?
8. Cluster concepts and form groups to leave the main direction open for discourse and bundle specific solution aspects.
9. Let groups elaborate on the concepts in a cluster and produce a few quality
   solutions: Quality is best achieved by putting different minds together.
10. Demand a clear strategy how to continue with these concepts, including
    system design, success factors and stakeholders to be integrated into further
    work. Without this, it is rather likely that the initial enthusiasm is washed
    away in everyone's everyday workload and little will happen to realize the
    innovation.
11. Determine a "caretaker" who will make sure that anything will happen at all.

Considerations on success and sense, again: Have they now been achieved?
However ingenious a concept and system design may be, it will never be successful nor produce any sense unless it is available for the intended purpose to the

respective target group(s) and is attractive to the users. The latter should by and large have been assured due to the preparatory work described above. However, the solution must still be accessible and affordable.

The availability of a solution means that it will have to be produced, distributed, and that its maintenance has to be assured in an appropriate scale, depending on the scope of potential application. All of this needs to be compatible with existing economic and social systems: In our project for example, the elderly people must be able to buy, rent, or be otherwise given or granted access to the Elisa system; a prototype that demonstrates effect but never reaches larger scale production is little more than just another showcase from just another research project.

Summary: the nature of innovation and the Holistic Innovation process
On the basis of the above discussion we hope that the reasoning of core elements of the Holistic Innovation methodology sketched before becomes clearer. We would like to point out again especially:

- The usefulness of a preparatory "thinking ahead future" which will also briefly be discussed in the chapter "Targeting: How We Defined a Project that Makes a Difference".
- The TargetVision summarizing the "sense" of the project and the interests of stakeholders.
- The exploration of the context system and the core functions—among these the intensive work on user motivations and interests—helping to understand and embed the task at stake.
- The concept development being positioned later than usual in innovation processes.
- The necessity not to forget the system design, integrating the concept into its environment.
- The product development and distribution concerns, making sure that a great solution will in fact create an effect on an appropriate scale.

More information on this topic can be found in (Moritz 2009), unfortunately only in German. And Innovationsmanufaktur will continue to work on these methodological aspects, always interested in productive discourse. Contact us!

References

Moritz, E.F.: Holistische Innovation. Konzept, Methodik und Beispiele. Springer, Heidelberg (2009)
Moritz, E.F., Ruth, K.: Ressourcen in Netzwerken – zur Chemie, Biologie, Physik und Metaphysik von Kooperation. In: Moldaschl, M. (ed.) Verwertung immaterieller Ressourcen. Rainer Hampp Verlag, München, Mering (2007)
Schumpeter, J.A.: The Theory of Economic Development. 13th Printing 2007. Transaction Publishers, New Brunswick (1934)

Targeting: How We Defined a Project that Makes a Difference

Martin Strehler and Eckehard Fozzy Moritz

1 Executive Summary

This chapter explains in theory, but much more so in practice, how we came up with the project idea for SI-Screen/Elisa, and why we were confident that we could develop a product that would make a difference for the user and become successful on the market.

2 Main Results

In all innovation work, there are different options for defining successful innovation projects. To give some examples:

- You can start by having an idea, then realize and optimize it, develop a business plan and hope that the product will be successful. Even though widely spread, this is certainly neither the most probable nor the most efficient way to success.
- According to the Holistic Innovation methodology, it would make much more sense to conceive a socially relevant system aspect of the future, e.g. the social interaction of the elderly, create a creative synergy of functions to be performed considering boundary conditions and utilizing innovation enablers, all filtered according to stakeholder interest. This means more work at the beginning, but usually saves a lot of resources and time later on, and moreover ensures a higher likelihood of success.
- Publically funded projects usually still demand a different approach: The general topic area is given, as are the expectations and boundary conditions in terms of predefined results, use of resources, and the integration of partners. Thus, in a

M. Strehler (✉) · E. F. Moritz
Innovationsmanufaktur GmbH, Munich, Germany
e-mail: ms@innovationsmanufaktur.com

E. F. Moritz (ed.), *Assistive Technologies for the Interaction of the Elderly*,
Advanced Technologies and Societal Change, DOI: 10.1007/978-3-319-00678-9_2,
© Springer International Publishing Switzerland 2014

15

Table 1 SI-Screen/Elisa consortium

Project partner	Organisation type	Country
Innovationsmanufaktur GmbH (former SportKreativWerkstatt)	Company (SME)	Germany
Brainware GmbH	Company (SME)	Germany
Universität der Bundeswehr München	University	Germany
Federació d'Associacions de Gent Gran de Catalunya	End User Organisation	Spain
Helios	Company (SME)	Italy
Instituto de Biomecánica de Valencia	Research Institute	Spain
Porsche Design Studio	Company	Austria
Servicios de Teleasistencia, S.A	Company	Spain
Tioman & Partners SL	Company (SME)	Spain
VIOS Medien GmbH	End User Organisation	Germany

more or less rigid frame, depending on the judging institutions and experts, you have to make most of all of this for innovation success.

The last example describes the point of origin of our SI-Screen/Elisa project. A call for proposals asked for "ICT based solutions for advancement of social interaction of elderly people". We needed to produce a project proposal that would integrate partners from at least three European countries, cost a couple of million euros, sounds promising in terms of result and market viability, and shows technical challenge and likelihood and methodology of solution. Yes, take it or leave it.

We took it. What we came up with was a proposal that promised to create a new user-oriented social interaction tool that would enable elderly people to stay or get in touch with family, friends and the neighborhood, and which helps finding and participating in local activity, health and wellbeing offers. The partner constellation we could set up for this project was truly unique, combining competences, experiences and a good reputation from four European countries. In fact, we are sure that the selection of partners did not only help us get the project granted, but also to create the great project we can present in this book (Table 1).

3 Storyline

In spring 2008, we first heard of a new abbreviation: AAL. Nowadays, Ambient Assisted Living is in large parts of the population still something unheard-of whereas it has become a very well-known term in areas like microelectronics, smart living, and demographical change or in the EU research funding scene.

Shortly after the first AAL JP call was released in 2008, the Innovations-manufaktur tried to find partners in the area of "prevention and management of chronic conditions of elderly people". Unfortunately, after coordinating and writing half of the proposal our Italian consortium leader turned out to be ineligible. In the following weeks we searched for ways to reintegrate him but we did not find a reasonable way and the whole project idea was abandoned.

But we were ready for the second call topic with the ambition not to fail again and to hand in a decent proposal and therefore we wanted to keep the reigns in Innovationsmanufaktur's hands this time. When the topic "ICT based solutions for advancement of social interaction of elderly people" was announced we knew that a Holistic Innovation approach combined with early user involvement could make a difference if we could succeed in finding a strong idea and the right partners. Experience had already shown us that the "not invented here" problem was not to be neglected. This means that approaching potential partners with a completed idea very often makes them skeptic because they had had no part in the origination of that idea. However, neither is it easy to convince potential partners to join a consortium without having a first idea of the work to be done.

Many AAL projects are technology-oriented but we took the possibility to start our project the way we think innovations should happen: With the needs of the users in mind, regardless of any technological constraints! After a first internal brainstorming and a few phone calls to (elderly) parents and their friends, two main objectives emerged. First, somehow having access to the internet and being part of this new world and second, easily keeping in touch with friends and family. Today, both these interests are contained in the term "social media" but only some years ago at the conception of Elisa, that phenomenon was still only emerging.

A midsize screen

The smartphone was still very young but already showed extraordinary growth and sales figures. Unfortunately, the devices were still very complex and the small displays were not likely to attract elderly people. Their understanding of a useful technology was dominated by the TV with its big screen and very easy usability. But there was also a new product that seemed to mesh very well with the needs of senior citizens: the digital picture frame. It was very easy to use; you just had to switch it on, insert a flash drive or photo card and seniors could enjoy something that they really appreciate—pictures of family and friends. This was still the time before the iPad was released and we envisioned something very similar: a device that had a big enough display for elderly people to easily consume information and content.

The first ideas

The simplest vision we thought of was a slideshow with friends and family on the screen, stimulating elderly people to get in contact with their friends just by touching the picture in the slideshow to start a video call. A more advanced feature to keep senior citizens up to date about their surroundings was the idea of providing them with information from different social networks (Fig. 1).

But we also wanted a very easy way for elderly people to become active and get in touch with friends and relatives beyond phone calls. As a first idea for an easy interaction we thought of rotating contacts on the one side of the screen and a list

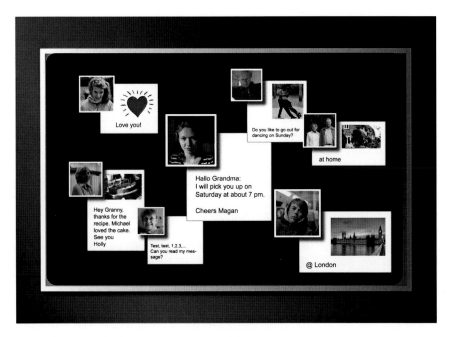

Fig. 1 First ideas of Elisa: a window to the social networks

of possible activities on the other side. Elements from both sides were supposed to be dragged into a personal calendar, thus automatically generating messages to other screens or social networks requesting to do joint activities (Fig. 2).

Visionary partners for a visionary idea

With our first vision of a new interaction screen we contacted our colleagues from the Universität der Bundeswehr München in order to discuss the idea and its feasibility. After bringing arguments from the user needs side together with the technical perspectives we agreed on integrating existing social media channels instead of trying to compete with them directly. We quickly found partners in Spain and Germany for the user-centered development approach and in both countries revived old contacts and established new ones. The most difficult task: finding a European producer who could develop tablet PCs—which actually were not yet invented. After a few weeks we had contacted quite a few hardware manufacturers, but there were two major problems: We could find only one European company in the Smartphone business and for all other companies (we spoke with e.g. Bang and Olufsen, Kodak, Archos) the promised success in tablet PCs was even less obvious. So in the end, we had to start the project without a technological developer in the consortium. At first, we thought this would be a major problem, but in retrospective, it turned out to be rather positive: In the meantime, enough tablet producers have entered the market that we can choose the best technology available and brand it

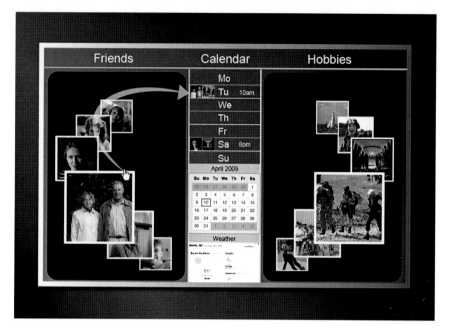

Fig. 2 First ideas of Elisa: an interaction tool

with the Elisa coating and software. Even if we had had a technology hardware producer they (and therefore our product) would have had to compete with giants like Apple or Samsung and we would have been restricted to a technology chosen three years ago.

Even better than a technology producer, we found in Porsche Design Studio a visionary partner who got involved in this very innovative development and who could upgrade the product by adapting the hardware chassis to the special needs of best agers and bringing in values like very high quality and puristic, timeless design associated with the brand Porsche and Porsche Design.

A strong proposal without too much predetermination
How could we write a convincing project proposal and still leave room for innovation and enhancement during the project process? That was one of our key concerns. Sure, in every research and development (R&D) proposal you have to have a sound idea and very good and complementary partners. But as a lot of money is requested by the team, many details have to be fixed in advance in order to convince the funding authorities of a well-calculated budget. With a very good idea, partners that believed in that idea and aided in the proposal writing and last but not least some quite good figures that indicated that there was a big market evolving, we could convince the international experts to grant the funding support for this project despite not being overly detailed about the concrete outcome.

That is how the SI-Screen/Elisa story started—with the focus on the needs, wishes and perspectives of elderly people and with us trying to set up not a technology-driven but a user need driven project, which has the potential to make a difference in the communication and social activity behavior of every elderly person. In the SI-Screen/Elisa project, the ICT should work for the user, not vice versa.

User Groups and Characteristics: How We Described the User Groups

Stefanie Erdt, Stephan Biel, Javier Ganzarain, Eckehard Fozzy Moritz and Ute Vidal Cabello

1 Executive Summary

As the target group of the SI-Screen/Elisa project—the elderly—is quite heterogeneous, we address in this chapter the question of how to best approach an in-depth understanding of this group and its needs and wishes. We started by creating a novel typology according to the two descriptors of "degree of social integration" and "technical affinity". After identifying the five types of Bon Vivant, Familizer, Shy Guy, Snoopy and Social Animal as our core reference types due to their low to middle technical affinity and their middle to high social activity, we proceeded by creating "personas" with real backstories for every type. This was needed to help all partners in the project to keep in view the future customers and their wishes and needs during the whole design process. Finally, all this was condensed into three in-depth users' stories thus rendering the end users' needs, environments and intercultural differences as visible and understandable as possible.

2 Main Results

The main result of this chapter is a novel typology of elderly people (Fig. 1). Even though various typologies of elderly people already exist, a new typology had to be developed especially for Elisa to correctly identify and describe those groups of

S. Erdt (✉) · E. F. Moritz
Innovationsmanufaktur GmbH, Munich, Germany
e-mail: se@innovationsmanufaktur.com

S. Biel · J. Ganzarain
Tioman & Partners SL, Barcelona, Spain

U. Vidal Cabello
VIOS Medien GmbH, Gröbenzell, Germany

E. F. Moritz (ed.), *Assistive Technologies for the Interaction of the Elderly*,
Advanced Technologies and Societal Change, DOI: 10.1007/978-3-319-00678-9_3,
© Springer International Publishing Switzerland 2014

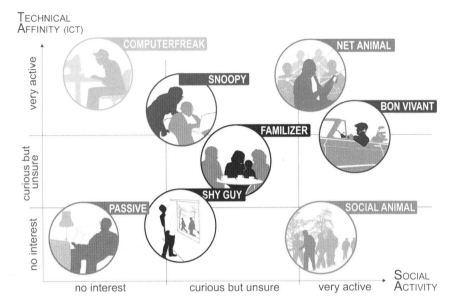

Fig. 1 Elisa typology

elderly that would benefit most from an innovation aimed at improving their social interaction with new technological solutions. The new typology was also used to direct development efforts and user integration activities to best serve the needs and wants of the user groups.

We defined eight possible profiles of people (Bon Vivant, Computer Freak, Familizer, Net Animal, Passive, Shy Guy, Snoopy and Social Animal), taking into account the amount of their social activity and their familiarity with technology.

3 Storyline

Why did we need a new typology?

So there we were: In the first big project meeting we had detailed our joint TargetVision as "to create a new economically, socially and culturally sustainable social interaction tool that enables elderly people to easily stay or get in touch with existing and new people of interest and which helps to find and participate in accessible local activities, health and wellbeing offers." As can easily be seen, most of the functionalities we wanted to realize were directly related to the ominous "elderly", their interests, habits, even their cultural imprint. But who exactly were these elderly? The more we tried to understand them, the more we realized that this is all but a homogeneous group; especially not one that could reasonably be described with a simple mix of single parameters like age, social status, and/or degree of education. Such a description might have been easy, but we needed something useful, not something easily done.

Our approach to that issue started with the following question: Is it possible to define, and then describe, groups, "types", of elderly that show similarities with regard to our innovation task and hence could serve to define requirements and constitute power groups for user integration? Thus, we found a suitable means to our end: the definition of so-called milieus (e.g. Sinus Milieus (http://www.sinus-institut.de/en)). But the traditional classifications of elderly people mostly refer to their health status (studying aspects such as frailty, autonomy, disability etc.), chronological data (age, gender etc.) or data about their lifecycle (when did they retire, when did the children leave the nest etc.). These classifications were not ideally suited to this project. Thus, we did not find any descriptions of milieus that met our demands and so we had to establish our own milieus, or types.

How did we create the typology?

All of this really started on a nice rooftop in Barcelona. In a small discussion round between Tioman & Partners and Innovationsmanufaktur, we tried to find descriptors for the axes that would span our ground field for the types, and provisionally filled it with what we knew from prior projects, other studies, and experiences in our project so far. As first guess, we used "degree of social integration", and "technical affinity" as descriptors, and identified eight types to which we assigned tentative names. It all seemed very plausible, but was of course not at all substantiated, hence not really useful yet.

This was the right time to pass on the ball to all project partners responsible for the end user integration. To help develop the picture further, the next step was to find a more detailed definition of the key parameters we had chosen as descriptors. The following aspects were fixed:

• personality and attitude to life: common characteristics, lifestyle, common behavioral denominator,
• social engagement and attitude towards society: social activity, responsibility towards society (person receives/gives support), social activities (place, time, level of participation),
• preferred leisure activities: public events/self-organized activities, appointment/ communication strategy, place, time, level of participation,
• number and quality of social contacts: distribution of family or friends, household composition, average amount of social contacts,
• technical affinity and attitude towards technology: use of ICT (frequency, purpose, concerns and motivations, experience level, skills), preferred way of communicating (face-to-face, phone, email, others).

Now, as we had formed the framework, we started to fill in the "flesh and bones" in the detailed description of our types Bon Vivant, Computer Freak, Familizer, Net Animal, Passive, Shy Guy, Snoopy and Social Animal. In doing so, it proved to be very helpful that some of the partners already had very close professional and personal contacts to our target group: having real persons in mind made it easy to paint a vivid portrait of every type. To condense the characteristic essence into a short form, we additionally created a slogan for each type (see Table 1).

After the typology definition and the focus groups we finally created "personas" with real backstories for every type in order to help all partners in the project to keep in view the future customers and their wishes and needs during the whole design process. The personas are: "Enjoying Sylvia" (Bon Vivant), "Caring Caren" (Familizer), "Juan the Cosmopolite" (Net Animal), "Demanding Martin" (Passive), "Shy Maria" (Shy Guy), "Curious Kurt" (Snoopy) and "Active Daisy" (Social Animal).

Explaining our typology and the most relevant types

Now we had to think about our core target group: Which types would benefit most from the future product Elisa? We selected the Bon Vivant, Familizer, Shy Guy, Snoopy and Social Animal types as reference because of their low to middle technical affinity and their middle to high social activity. Additionally, we chose the Net Animal type in order to gain feedback from elderly people with a high social activity and technical affinity level as a comparison to the less involved user types. Moreover, they could thus also improve their social activities and their use of ICT technology. The technology to be developed itself could be also useful for the Net Animals because it could introduce new services or functionalities. The type Computer Freak had to be excluded because of its high experience in new technologies—a Computer Freak will not experience much added value through Elisa. Moreover, it would be very hard to motivate the Computer Freak type to have more social interaction, a trait he/she by the way shares with the Passive type. The latter was excluded as well, as it will not be interested in handling new technical devices, and was also considered a decreasing type in the following generations of elderly people. Thus, the types Bon Vivant, Familizer, Shy Guy, Snoopy and Social Animal form our core target group, since Elisa has the potential to improve their social integration and to remove barriers as far as the use of ICT is concerned.

In Table 1, the five selected types are presented shortly according to their personality, social and leisure activities and technical affinity.

For what did we use these types?

The definition of the types helped us to understand the differences between the identified groups regarding their social interaction and focus and which social activities each of them are willing to perform.

As a next step, we formed focus groups in Germany and Spain, on the one hand to get a detailed insight into the users' behavior and needs; and on the other hand to prove the validity of our typology. We decided to run five focus groups in Germany and Spain, respectively. A focus group is a qualitative methodology that consists of a carefully planned conversation, designed to obtain information on a specific subject, in a permissive, non-direct atmosphere. The topics addressed during the focus groups were:

Table 1 Short description of the five selected Elisa types

Personality	Social and leisure activities	Technical affinity
Bon Vivant "Now I have time to enjoy my life!"		
Modern, liberal and spontaneous person	Likes to enjoy life to the fullest with like-minded people	Uses ICT to get information and to organize her/his leisure activities
Culturally educated and interested	Active and pleasant lifestyle	
Trendy and up to date, appearance matters	Dining out in fancy restaurants, wellness in luxury spas, travelling, learning languages, music, theatre, shopping, sports and parties	Technically well equipped with "hip" communication and entertainment media devices
		Knows about social networks but prefers to communicate directly
Familizer: "My family is my life!"		
Conservative and traditional person	Family and close friends are the center of her/his life	Is not familiar with the computer and the internet, needs others to help out with technical tasks
Open-minded as well as responsible	Enjoys social groups and family activities	
Positive attitude towards life, talkative and devoted to supporting others	Playing cards and board games, gardening, regular visits to pubs, honorary social work, learning languages, travelling and outdoor activities	Uses mostly traditional communication devices like telephone and cell phone, sometimes e-mail
		Doesn't know what exactly a virtual network is and is not interested due to a preference for face-to-face communication
Shy Guy: "I would try but I am afraid of breaking it!"		
Unconfident and timid person who needs support in many areas of life	Only few contacts, including close friends and neighbors, fixed on family	Likes to use ICT to watch pictures of family and friends
Quiet, shy and indecisive	Eager for companionship, but little individual initiative	Uses only traditional devices, fearing to break devices or do something wrong
Traditional, afraid of changes	Activities at home like reading, watching TV, gardening	Frightened about breach of privacy in virtual social networks
Snoopy: "Ok, I'll try this!"		
Conservative, traditional and pragmatic person	Close contacts to like-minded friends and closest family, contact to relatives reduced to obligating events	Uses ICT mainly to get information, to communicate and to organize daily life and leisure activities
Curious with multi-layered interests	Very active lifestyle, enjoys various activities	Only few but functional electronic devices
Critical but open-minded attitude	Travelling, honorary work, political engagement, theatre, reading consumer magazines	Knows about virtual social networks, but is not sure if they are useful

(continued)

Table 1 (continued)

Personality	Social and leisure activities	Technical affinity
Social Animal: "I love spending time with my friends!"		
Very social and active person with a variety of interests	Close contacts to family and friends	Not really interested in technical devices, uses only necessary and useful ones
Engaged, helpful person with a big social conscience	Active and socially/ environmentally engaged lifestyle	Communicates by phone, cell phone or sometimes e-mail
Open-minded, but not uncritical	Loves to be on the road and to meet friends, cultural and social activities, outdoor activities in the group, chatting	Sees no real added value in virtual social networks, prefers real life interactions

- How elderly people interact socially,
- Methods used to relate to other people,
- Level of use of Internet by elderly people,
- Design trends for the Elisa tool,
- Level of interest in purchasing an Elisa tool.

Due to the validity of our typology, the results of the focus groups were very gratifying: Our hypothetical descriptions hit the mark in almost all aspects and we had to correct only small details.

Showing the differences between Germany and Spain
The intercultural differences between the results of the discussion groups of both countries have also been analyzed regarding the following issues:

- How do elderly people interact socially (motives, interests and activities)?
- Which methods are used to interact with other people?
- How high is the level of Internet usage by elderly people?

Concerning the "how" of the elderly people's social interaction with other people, we firstly collected motives and interests defining their relationships. Secondly, we had a look at the activities the elderly employ daily in their relationships with other people. It has to be noted, however, that our conclusions were reached from a reduced sample of users, and therefore may indicate trends but have to be considered cautiously (Table 2).

Intercultural similarities and differences: analysis and conclusions
All this information was condensed into an analysis which showed that, actually, there are a lot of common aspects shared by both populations, such as main concerns about specific health topics (for instance blood pressure and overweight), or main worries regarding the use of/approach to ICT (i.e. safety or user-friendliness).

As regards the differences, our research showed that the Spanish in general were more family-oriented whereas the German elderly had stronger technological links.

Table 2 Social interaction: intercultural differences

How elderly people interact socially: motives and interests in their social relationships	
Spain	*Germany*
Meeting people with the same interests	Contact to other persons (in a broader sense)
Having company (not feeling lonely)	Help or support others
Enjoying the activity itself	Do something they always wanted to do (new challenges, learning something new)
Talking (be able to unburden themselves by telling their problems to others) (Shy Guy)	Longing to be integrated (Shy Guy)

How elderly people interact socially: activities performed daily to interact with other people	
Spain	*Germany*
Meet family/friends for having lunch/dinner	Meet family for special family events (birthdays, jubilees, holidays....)
Travelling (only the Spanish Bon Vivant might also travel alone)	Travelling (all, in general, might also travel alone)
Help is family/relatives oriented (the Bon Vivant does not help)	Help is family/relatives oriented (in general)
Volunteering (only the Snoopy)	Honorary work (on their own) (not the Net Animal)
Mostly more passive/non sportive (Musical, concerts, watching football, reading, painting, bingo, cards) and some outside activities (gardening, going out for a walk)	Activities similar to the Spanish activities and also more active ones (indoors like swimming, dancing, playing instruments and table-tennis and outdoors in natural environments like hiking, cycling, Nordic walking, shooting and even risky ones, e.g. skiing)

Approaches for interaction with other people	
Spain	*Germany*
Organizing mostly by telephone followed by a personal visit (to decide whether to participate or not)	Organizing mostly by email (all but Shy Guy (meets mainly in person or calls people))
Mobile phone (basic ones to make/receive calls and text messages). Some of the elderly even take pictures and use other services	Using mobile phone when they are on the road, in cases of emergency (security, safety) or to be available
The groups considered initially to be more technologically advanced use the Internet to communicate with relatives and friends	Using modern communication and information media dependent on the subject of communication and also adapted to the communication partner. They even send handwritten letters to special persons for special occasions

(continued)

Table 2 (continued)

Level of Internet use by elderly people	

Spain

Opinion

- Good, convenient, interesting, but if you are unfamiliar with it, you are isolated from the rest of society and if you do not use it you will be left behind (it is indispensable today)
- Limits real interaction/social relationships
- Creates fear, insecurity (risks, privacy problems, isolation)

Utilisation

- To communicate with relatives and distant friends
- To see photos/videos
- To make doctor's, tax office and test appointments

Problems

- Lack of time/perseverance
- Limits interactions/experiences
- Lack of (methodology/experience) training (no patience)
- Too many unneeded and unused functions
- Finding someone to show them properly
- Fear of various aspects of usage (breaking it, getting lost while surfing, not much privacy (getting exposed in social nets), mistrust, ridicule, possibility of fraud, spam, etc.)

Opportunities

- Ease (also voice recognition) and simplicity
- It should not encourage isolation
- Improve the way of teaching
- Having the time and motivation to learn
- If a person can communicate with voice and image, then there is a feeling of warmth

Germany

- Some things are cheaper, faster, more up to date and it offers comprehensive information (e.g. evaluation of hotels)
- Makes it easier to communicate (with family, former students and colleagues), but you stay at home more
- Cannot try selected products (such as clothes) but can see them (e.g. hotels), offers warranty

- Online-shopping and banking (no restricted opening hours)

- Lack of clarity/different structures are confusing
- Complexity of menus (structure and language), user manuals and device operation (adjustability, legibility (also AGBs) and size of buttons). Problems finding the right words for the search engines
- Tech development too fast, need help with PC trouble
- Too much "blah-blah" conversation over the mobile phone
- More critical with safety/data abuse, advertising, speed, waste of time (Facebook)
- No direct awareness
- No personal advice/service online
- No going out

- Easy, safe, reliable (also seal of quality) and suited to their needs
- Support for their computer problems, e.g. 24/7 hotlines, remote maintenance, installation support (or no installation needed), seniors-help-seniors, classes for beginners and advanced users

Table 3 Ambient setting structure

Structure	Description
Where	Place where the action happens
Aim of the action	Why and for what is this action carried out?
Primary user, protagonist	Who is the user of Elisa?
Secondary user, secondary actors	Who interacts with the primary user? Could for example be family, friends, and carers
Assumptions and preconditions	Assumptions and preconditions required to understand the scenario
Application/software	Application required to use Elisa
Technology	Device or devices required for the action in question
Other non-technological hardware	Complementary non-tech hardware to make Elisa sexier, more usable, more comfortable to transport. For example cases, frames, ...
Related services	What services should be provided by Elisa in order to meet user needs?
Unrelated services	Services that will not be provided by Elisa as they are out of its scope
Process	Steps needed to develop the ambient settings (only developed for the first use of Elisa)
Service payer	Who will pay the service?
Service buyer or purchaser	Who will decide on or regulate the purchase of the service?

The Spanish elderly met with their family on an everyday basis, for example during lunch on weekends, offered mutual support, and undertook at least some activities every week. The Germans, however, rather met during leisure time and offered support on special occasions rather than on "normal" days. This became especially obvious in case of the "Shy Guy" type. In Spain she or he was nonetheless mostly well connected to the family network, whereas in Germany, the "Shy Guy" type consisted mainly of women who had no financial security and very little contact to their families. The factor "use of technology" disclosed a smaller difference between the two countries than we expected at the beginning. The differences we did find were mostly due to the corresponding external factors such as the fact that broadband internet is not as much developed in rural Spain as it is in Germany. Also, access to the internet is cheaper in Germany than in Spain.

Ambient settings and use case scenarios
In order to make these types and intercultural differences more visible and understandable to the developers of the future product Elisa, and for the reflection on which hardware best fits the Elisa concept, which services should be considered as well as in which conditions, environments, scenarios Elisa could be used, we also developed concrete ambient settings and user stories for each of the types in Germany and Spain.

First, a common structure was defined for the ambient settings, which is shown in Table 3.

The next step in the project was the definition of an agreement on one ambient setting that will be the input for the development team and for the visualization of the use scenarios. The ambient setting selected was "Elisa at home" which covers more of the elderly, meets the needs of the target end user group better and combines the three Elisa functionalities: be inspired, get information and communicate (see Functions: How We Understood and Realized Functions of Real Importance to Users). It also makes use of the best technology for Elisa, a 10-inch tablet PC (for the selection process of the tablet type, see Evaluation: How We Tested and Optimized Elisa) with an Elisa frame.

Then, based on the end user requirements and the focus group reports from Germany and Spain, user stories were developed in detail to explore the social relationship of elderly people and how the "elderly interaction and service assistant" (Elisa) fosters social interaction and well-being at an old age. Following the practice of user-centered design, we created personas, fictional characters with all the characteristics of elderly persons (primary stakeholders), and their goals and motivations that correspond to real-life situations and the ambient settings in which Elisa and the corresponding functionalities would be used. Personas are important to understand the possible problems and difficulties of elderly people and the actual needs of the target group.

Our user stories: putting faces to the Elisa scenarios
The results of these efforts have been combined into three user stories. Each user story represents a different persona according to the socio-technological typology. "Eva Keppler" in Munich, Germany is a Social Animal: She is a very social and active person with a variety of interests, has close contacts to family and friends and little or no experience with computers or other technical devices. "Pepe Martínez Molins", who lives in Barcelona, Spain, is a Familizer, a conservative and traditional person, his family and close friends are the centre of his life and he has some experience with computers and the Internet. "Christobal Orts Verdú" is a Bon Vivant who enjoys life in Valencia, Spain, with like-minded people and uses ICT to organise his leisure activities. All three are also friends with each other in order to facilitate simulating interaction between them, as can also be seen in their social interaction flows that have been included in Communication. Below you can find the whole user story of Eva Keppler and a short excerpt from the stories of Pepe and Christobal.

Eva Keppler's Story: how Eva Keppler masters the challenge of Diabetes and more…
Eva Keppler, a 69-year-old woman, is living with her 70-year-old friend Alex in an apartment in the suburbs of Munich. Both of them are retired. She is divorced from Klaus (72), has a daughter (Anna, 42), a son (Peter, 40), two grandchildren (Julia, 17 and Markus, 15) and a lot of friends. She usually goes to a local sports center to practice physical activities (Pilates, yoga, swimming…). Eva is very happy about Elisa, a new tablet computer for people who are not familiar with computers and the Internet. A personal assistant very comfortable to use, that helps establish contact to people and groups sharing the same interests, provides well-founded,

reliable health information and informs her about latest activities and news in town. Moreover, Elisa is adaptable to each of Eva's and Alex's individual needs so they can both share the same device and still retain their personal contacts and receive individual information adapted to their personal profiles. Best of all, Eva and Alex do not have to configure Elisa at all. Instead, her son Peter, who is living in Berlin, is able to setup and maintain Elisa for Eva and Alex by remote.

Elisa was recommended to Eva by her friend Jürgen (70) from the sports center, who gave an introduction to the system. And Eva was so convinced by the easiness and joyfulness that she decided to buy her own Elisa tablet PC.

At her recent medical check-up she was informed that she is suffering from Diabetes mellitus Type II. Apart from the advices of her doctor, she is eager to know more about Diabetes and what helped other people her age to live with this disease. Thus, she uses Elisa to read more information on this health topic. While she is reading an article, Elisa presents her with additional information on self-help groups near her home in Munich. Being curious about one of the self-help groups, Eva is shown not only the phone contact and address of that Diabetes group, but also all recommendations of others, when the next meeting takes place and that it is free of charge. Eva tips on the displayed phone number to use Elisa's telephone feature and call the contact person of the Diabetes group to announce her visit. For this, Elisa uses her landline telephone.

After Eva's first visit to the Diabetes self-help group, she regularly joins the group meetings, as she feels very comfortable and finds the exchange of experience with other members regarding Diabetes very helpful. She becomes friends with Ruth, a woman five years older than her, and they also meet outside the Diabetes group.

Meanwhile, Elisa "learns" about Eva's interest in Diabetes and provides Eva with relevant up-to-date health information articles concerning this disease. Eva is very inspired by the latest Diabetes article offered by Elisa, so she invites Ruth to read the article by just selecting Ruth's picture from her personal contact list. Ruth is also very curious about the new Diabetes treatment that promises to ease their lives. Therefore, she in turn comments on the article, thus providing written feedback to Eva and they begin a cheerful discussion about this treatment.

Some weeks later, while reading Elisa news during her daily coffee break, Eva is informed by Elisa that the "National Diabetes Days" will take place in Munich at the beginning of next month. They will include different activities like lectures of specialists, nutrition workshops and regional offers. Eva wants to inform the other group members and, as she already uses the invitation feature of Elisa quite often, she recommends this activity to all other members of her Diabetes self-help group by adding the whole group to the article. All the group members using Elisa get the notification instantly while everybody else receives the activity information by e-mail. Eva's son Peter helped her create the contact group with all its members remotely, but she thinks she will be able to do it herself the next time.

Pepe Martínez Molins' story: how Pepe stays in contact with his loved ones and more...

Pepe is a 70 years old man living with his wife María (67) in a flat in the center of Barcelona...

...A few days after a neighbor told Pepe and María about Elisa, they really bought their own Elisa tablet PC. It was very easy to start the first time as their daughter could support them remotely from Sitges. First of all, they contacted their grandson in Sydney and they were very happy because they could finally see all the lovely photos and follow his current activities via his personal blog. Pepe and María were really delighted with Elisa, its easiness and the possibilities it was offering them, like staying informed about the lives of their family members (small-talk, pictures etc.), follow their activities (reading their blogs and twitter accounts) and even plan some activities together (a family dinner or visit a new restaurant, an excursion). All of this was very easy due to a specific group Pepe made for this purpose with his daughter's support...

Cristobal Orts Verdú's story: how Cristobal closed a page of his life and opened a window to new horizons...

Cristobal is 65 years old and lives in one of the modern areas of Valencia. Over the last years he has experienced a lot of changes...

...When his daughter reads about a new device called Elisa, she recognizes it as a perfect solution to a lot of his needs, and decides to give it to Cristobal as a birthday present. As part of the gift, she would do not only the first installation of the device but also carry out all the administrative tasks that Cristobal himself finds so "boring".

Cristobal really likes Elisa because now it is really delightful to be updated regularly on 15M, a Spanish social movement, and their activities. It is also quite easy to stay in contact with his old friend Pepe in Barcelona, who owns an Elisa device as well. Last week for example Pepe informed Cristobal via Elisa about a jazz concert in Barcelona with an artist he had wanted to see live on stage for years. Spontaneously, Cristobal decided to travel to Barcelona, see the concert and enjoy a day together with Pepe at the beach talking about his future plans and the good old days...

User Involvement: How We Integrated Users into the Innovation Process and What We Learned from It

Ricard Barberà-Guillem, Nadia Campos, Stephan Biel, Stefanie Erdt, Javier Gámez Payá, Javier Ganzarain and Ute Vidal Cabello

1 Executive Summary

It is the general message of the whole book that the users and future buyers of a product or service have to take part in the innovation process from the strategic phase to the go to market stage. In this chapter, we will describe how we integrated the elderly and their needs, values, expectancies and preferences into the Elisa innovation activities with specific tools and methodologies. We grouped these methodologies into three main areas: (1) definition of the problem; (2) analysis of needs and elaboration of specifications; and (3) test of the product.

A total number of 350 users aged 50+ participated in at least one of the tools used in the different stages of the Elisa development. The project began with quite an open target as described in Targeting: How We Defined a Project That Makes a Difference. Then, as the consortium gained a better understanding of elderly people (regarding ICT affinity and social interaction), we narrowed the focus down to the central part of the Elisa users' typologies. At the same time, the Elisa concept became increasingly detailed while we refined the technical specifications and functionalities.

R. Barberà-Guillem (✉) · N. Campos
Instituto de Biomecánica de Valencia, Valencia, Spain
e-mail: ricard.barbera@ibv.upv.es

S. Biel · J. Ganzarain
Tioman & Partners SL, Barcelona, Spain

S. Erdt · J. Gámez Payá
Innovationsmanufaktur GmbH, Munich, Germany

U. Vidal Cabello
VIOS Medien GmbH, Gröbenzell, Germany

E. F. Moritz (ed.), *Assistive Technologies for the Interaction of the Elderly*,
Advanced Technologies and Societal Change, DOI: 10.1007/978-3-319-00678-9_4,
© Springer International Publishing Switzerland 2014

2 Main Results

The success of the integration of the elderly users into the Elisa project has two main positive results. The first one relates to a satisfactory adaptation and use of the methodologies in an ICT environment with elderly persons. The second one refers to the number of ideas and recommendations from the users that were first incorporated into the concept and later into the different prototypes during the four-stage iterative user involvement development process.

3 Storyline

The TargetVision of the project was based on the following hypotheses, taken from the perspectives of the users:

- Many elderly people do not use social networking sites because access devices are generally not suited to their skills, abilities and preferences.
- A tool providing access to social networks in which the visual aspects are prioritized resulting in an easier and more intuitive navigation procedure will allow for greater adaptation by elderly persons.
- A flexible system allowing the incorporation of new technologies and future services will improve the viability of the whole system.
- The system will be more appealing to the elderly people if it integrates social and health services.

First, we needed to corroborate these hypotheses, and then systematically translate them into design criteria and specifications until reaching the final product. We walked this path with the users by means of objective, qualitative and quantitative techniques, based on the IBV approach of User Oriented Innovation (IOP) (Lahuerta 2010; Such 2010; Campos 2010).

Figure 1 shows all the methodologies used in SI-Screen/Elisa considering the areas of development of the project in which an intensive participation of the users is demanded. These areas are: the definition of the problem, the analysis of needs and elaboration of specifications and, finally, the validation of the product. These three areas are coherent with the IOP and USERFIT (Poulson et al. 1996) models, as well as consistent with the Holistic Innovation scheme (Fig. 1, Process: How We Structured an Innovation Project Towards Maximum Use Value) applied in this project. In the Elisa approach, users played a key role in defining the core functions of the product, assessing the advancement of the development (from concept to last demonstrator) and identifying some key aspects of the product in relation to the introduction to the market.

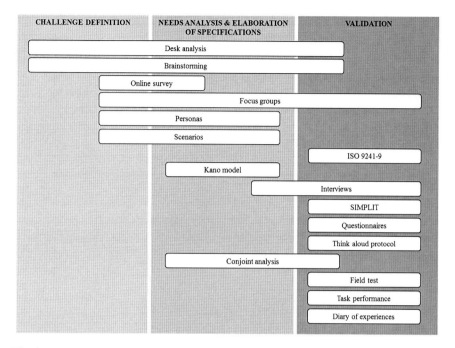

Fig. 1 Representation of the methodologies used to integrate the elderly persons in the SI-Screen/Elisa project

3.1 Definition of the Challenge

The definition of the challenge is clearly linked to the initial hypotheses and the goals to be achieved. On the one hand, we wanted to facilitate the access of elderly persons to the information society, often hampered by interfaces characterized by a lack of usability and excessive cognitive load. On the other hand, the technology should also facilitate social interaction and participation by taking into account activities offered in the users' close vicinity.

After an extensive literature review, an online survey was conducted among elderly people in Germany and Spain to further define the project approach. A total number of 232 elderly persons participated in this survey. This enabled us to define the TargetVision of the project as well as reach a deep understanding of elderly persons' "world" especially concerning ICT affinity and social interaction.

3.2 Analysis of Needs and Elaboration of Functions and Specifications

During the desk analysis, we found a lot of published information on the characterization of the elderly. The challenge was to translate this information into product requirements and then into technical specifications including the functionalities to be implemented in Elisa.

We began with a very open approach in order to avoid omitting important or relevant information. We then narrowed the scope until we obtained the core group functionalities. The first two steps, identification of the users' needs and translation into product requirements, were mainly user driven. The third step introduced the technology side of the problem with a very challenging translation of user requirements into product specifications. Taking into account these specifications and comparing them to current systems, we selected those with a high potential to evolve into groundbreaking system solutions.

Identifying the users' needs

As a first step, we collected as much information about the elderly and their actual and potential needs and wishes as possible. To this end, we employed the following tools: desk analysis, online survey, focus groups and experts' analysis.

The desk analysis together with the previous experience of the partners was the main input to establish the different types of elderly persons (see User Groups and Characteristics: How We Described the User Groups).

In the end, by summing up all the input from different sources we produced a workable list of users' needs, wishes, and functionalities to be developed. We grouped and prioritized the needs from an expert's point of view. In some cases, we (re)wrote them using a language close to the user, for example, one of the needs of the user was defined as "to stay in (or not to lose) contact, meeting and talking, to friends and family/relatives (nearby and far away). Including having company or interacting with people".

Translating the users' needs into requirements and technical specifications

Users' needs were only the first step to produce the technical specifications of the Elisa system. From the users' needs, we needed to move on to requirements, functionalities and specifications. One of the requirements was defined as "being an easy and simple tool, suited to the needs of elderly users"; paying attention to this requirement we identified and addressed the following questions:

1. What is the time required to understand and learn the use of the application?
2. What is the optimal size of the keyboard?
3. What are the recommended contrast values for the screen?
4. What is the optimal number of functionalities or features available in each screen or menu?
5. How long does it take to localize the information needed?
6. How difficult is it to localize that information on the system?

7. How do elderly users deal with technical terms and English words (if they are not English speakers)?
8. Do users understand the instruction manual?

Thus, we obtained a long list of requirements and functionalities but had too little time and resources to develop and implement all of them. Therefore, a selection and prioritization became necessary for which we applied the Kano model. This methodology allows the classification of functionalities into three main categories: basic ("must have"), performance ("should have") and excitement ("wow" factor). This classification takes into account factors such as required effort for implementation, degree of novelty and impact on the final product, or technical difficulty. In the final selection, a consensus had to be reached between the "social" and the "technical" partners balancing users' desires and technical implementation possibilities. Selected functionalities for Elisa were "be inspired", "communication" and "information", for example.

3.3 Test of the Product

During every development process, it is necessary to introduce elements of evaluation to ensure that the development is on the right track. In our case, this meant that we needed to answer to the following groups of questions:

- In relation to the functionalities of the system: Is the system answering to the interests/needs of the user? What can the user do with the system? Even better, what can the system do for the user?
- In relation to the accessibility and usability of the system: Can the user take advantage of the functionalities of the system? Alternatively, is it too difficult to use or to understand?
- In relation to the perception and the desire of purchase: Is the system appealing to the user? Is the user willing to own and use the Elisa system?

These questions are partially answered in this chapter during the scientific excursion. Specific aspects of users groups and needs are tackled in User Groups and Characteristics: How We Described the User Groups, while functionalities and design elements are shown in Functions: How We Understood and Realized Functions of Real Importance to Users and Design: How We Attempted to Attract Users in Optics, Haptics, and Ease of Utilization. Evaluation: How We Tested and Optimized Elisa details the results of the validation and how the system fulfilled the needs and desires of the elderly. Finally, more business-related aspects are explained in Business: How We Worked to Get Elisa into the Market and Share the Benefits.

Table 1 shows the type of tests applied to the different prototypes during the development of the project. Prototype 0, was just the tablet, prototype I a mock-up, prototype II a functional version, and prototype III a completely functional version ready to be used in a real home environment.

4 Scientific Excursion

At this point, we present a brief summary of the different methodologies and tools used during the project. We grouped them into three main categories: generic, qualitative and quantitative tools.

4.1 Generic Tools

Desk analysis
This technique consists of gathering and analyzing information already available in print or published on the internet, with the objective of identifying the critical points of current knowledge including substantive findings as well as theoretical and methodological contributions to a particular topic. Desk analysis is based on secondary sources and therefore does not entail any new or original experimental work.

In the framework of the SI-Screen/Elisa project, desk analysis was performed to identify information on the elderly already published in specific fields such as social interaction or technology affinity as well as in generic fields such as the sociodemographics of elderly persons, usability and accessibility of ICT devices or technology trends for people aged 50+. We reviewed documents such as ETSI EG 202 116 V1.2.2 (2009-03) *Human Factors (HF; Guidelines for ICT products and services; "Design for all")* or general statistics data published by Eurostat,[1] INE[2] or DESTATIS.[3]

Online survey
A survey is an investigation of the characteristics of a given population by means of collecting data from a sample of that population and estimating their characteristics by means of the systematic use of statistical methodology (UNECE 2000). The term "survey" covers any activity that collects or acquires statistical data. Included are censuses, sample surveys, the collection of data from administrative

---

[1] European Statistical Office http://epp.eurostat.ec.europa.eu/

[2] Instituto Nacional de Estadística (Spanish Statistical Office) http://www.ine.es/

[3] Statistisches Bundesamt (German Statistical Office) https://www.destatis.de/

Table 1 Prototype development and aspects evaluated

	Concept	Functionality	Accessibility and usability	Acceptance, perception, and purchase intention
Prototype 0			X	
Prototype I	X			X
Prototype II		X	X	X
Prototype III		X	X	X

records and derived statistical activities (Statistics 1998). A survey entails at least the following steps:

- Formulating the objectives,
- Creating the survey instruments,
- Testing the survey,
- Conducting the survey,
- Analyzing the results.

From October to December 2010, we performed an online survey in Germany and Spain with 317 participants on average aged 40+, 127 in Germany and 190 in Spain. The group of people aged 61–70 years was the most representative with 36 % of the participants. The survey was structured into four main areas: (1) demographical data, (2) leisure activities, (3) technical affinity, and (4) health and prevention. The main result of the survey was the verification and the production of a deeper understanding of the types and their respective characteristics.

4.2 Qualitative Tools

Brainstorming

Brainstorming is not a specific tool for the inclusion of elderly people, but rather a generic technique for group creativity during which efforts are made to find a conclusion for a specific problem by gathering a list of ideas spontaneously contributed by the members of the group. The underlying idea is that working as a group is more effective than working individually on generating new ideas or concepts, as well as finding solutions to existing problems. Today, the term "brainstorming" is usually used as a catch-all for various group ideation sessions.

In the SI-Screen/Elisa project, different traditional as well as innovative group ideation techniques were used to produce and share a common objective and to reach an agreement on the characteristics of the product and details of development. Brainstorming has also been used as part of the focus group discussions with elderly people.

Focus group (Jordan 2000; Poveda et al. 2003a)

By means of focus groups, individual subjectivities can be compared with a group description, and it also connects different perspectives, experiences and points of view at a qualitative and exploratory level. This method consists of a carefully planned conversation designed to obtain information on a specific subject in a permissive, non-directed atmosphere. The group is composed of a relatively small set of people, from six to eight, directed by an expert moderator in a relaxed, comfortable atmosphere with the purpose of knowing what the participants think, how they feel or what they know about the subject under discussion. The participants are selected based on uniformity regarding the subject being studied.

As regards the SI-Screen/Elisa project, we obtained by means of this methodology information on the way elderly people interact socially and their relationship (affinity or hostility) with technology. Based on these two central topics, we defined eight possible profiles of people, taking into account their greater or lesser degree of social activity and their familiarity with ICT (Functions: How We Understood and Realized Functions of Real Importance to Users). From these eight profiles, we selected five as the most interesting for the objectives of the project, namely: Bon Vivant, Familizer, Shy Guy, Snoopy and Social Animal. In total, ten focus groups took place, five in Germany and five in Spain.

Heuristic evaluation

Heuristic evaluations are one of the most informal methods of usability inspection in the field of human-computer interaction. They are used to identify usability problems in the user interface (UI) design. A heuristic evaluation specifically involves evaluators ("experts") examining the interface and judging its compliance with recognized usability principles (the "heuristics"). Often the heuristic evaluation is conducted in the context of use cases (typical user tasks), to provide the developers with feedback on the extent to which the interface is likely to be compatible with the intended users' needs and preferences. The simplicity of heuristic evaluation is its strongest point while the main criticism is the high influence of the knowledge of the expert reviewer(s) on the results (Poveda et al. 2003a, b; Wikipedia 2013).

We used heuristic evaluation in several phases of the development of Elisa, sometimes based on the previous experience of consortium partners and sometimes supported by a list of marked or preselected aspects (i.e. during the evaluation of prototypes one and two).

Interviews

The interview is a communication process which normally takes place between two people. The selection of the interviewee is usually based on their knowledge on the subject of study. In this process, the interviewer gets information from the interviewee directly. It is a formal conversation, with intentionality, objectives and a more or less defined format. When preparing the script of the interview we (Juriasti 2003):

- took into account the objectives of the research and the targeted population of the interview,
- moved from general to more specific questions,
- moved from less compromising to the most confidential questions,
- went from less relevant issues to the most central,
- went from the description of the facts to their interpretation.

In the framework of Elisa, we used this technique at different moments, the most important during the validation of the first prototype. We wrote a script beforehand in order to set the topics of the talks and fix the terms used to express the different concepts and ideas of the Elisa system. We paid special attention to ensure an "understandable" language. The objective of the interview was to get opinions on the concept, functions, hardware and graphical user interface. In addition to verbal explanations, we used images and videos to support the interview.

Personas

Personas are fictional characters based on in-depth descriptions of users (Pruitt and Grudin 2003) created to represent the different user types within a targeted demographic, attitude and/or behavior set who might use a site, brand or product in a similar way. These personas often represent the extreme members of a user group since designing for them will also include the more ordinary users (Cooper 2008). This methodology focuses the attention on aspects of design and use that other methods do not take into consideration. Personas can be used to start discussions related to the features of the products in question; trying to answer questions such as: "Would "Martin" use this feature?" The personas technique can also help the design team to generate and improve design ideas (Grudin and Pruitt 2002). The personas technique usually follows these steps (Nelsen 2007):

- Finding the users: The objective of this step is to get as much knowledge of the users as possible. We can use several sources, for example interviews, observations, or reports.
- Building a hypothesis: In this step, we focus on users in a certain context.
- Constructing personas: This step consists of putting "a face and a body" to the personas. This happens by means of the description of five areas: body, psyche, background, emotions and attitudes, and personal traits.

In Elisa, the main application and use value of the persona approach was to depict and thus make "vivid" the characters of the milieus created and selected. It helped to better understand and communicate the differences among the different user groups. It also helped to understand the heterogeneity and diversity of the users' lives and to focus on how to meet their actual needs.

Scenario building

Scenarios are widely used in product development. Designers intuitively place themselves in the user's position and try to forecast possible situations in which the user has problems or needs related to the use context; then they aim to produce solutions that cover those needs or problems. Scenarios provide examples of usage as an input for the design and can be used as input for evaluation (using scenarios in, for example, a focus group or interview). Scenarios are used in the "need identification, concept generation, design and communication" phases of the product development process (Hasdoğan et al. 2006) with the users and within the design team. This technique is similar to using personas except that greater emphasis is put on the tasks the users undertake. Personas are often part of (characters in) a scenario.

We used several scenarios or ambient settings to explore how Elisa performs in different environments of a prospective customer. For this purpose, we defined use case scenarios and analyzed their relevance for the Elisa end product. These scenarios were: first use, at home, on tour and in a public domain. To build each of the scenarios we described different components for them (see Table 7, User Groups and Characteristics: How We Described the User Groups).

Think aloud test (Jordan 2000)
In this technique, users express their thoughts while performing series of specific tasks, including free navigation. Users are asked to say what they are seeing, thinking, doing and feeling while doing the tasks. This allows the observers to understand the thought process of the user. A session can also be recorded on audio or video. The main advantage of this technique is that we can obtain a lot of information with a reduced number of users. On the other hand, users may tend to be more rational and want to "do well", avoiding expressions like "I like the design because it is sumptuous and I will be envied by all my neighbors".

We used this technique in Elisa during the validation of the second prototype in combination with the SIMPLIT methodology described below.

4.3 Quantitative Tools

ISO 9241-9 (2002) Evaluating Non-Keyboard Input devices
The ISO 9241-9 (2002) standard proposes a range of performance tests to evaluate the ergonomic requirements for non-keyboard input devices, in our case: tablet PCs. The focus of the standard is on measuring the accuracy of computer mice, joysticks, trackballs, pens, and touchscreens (Douglas et al. 1999; Soukoreff and MacKenzie 2004). Following this standard, we employed the proposed multi-direction tapping task and applied Fitts' law equation to compare the results of different tablet computers.

The main objective of using this technique in the project SI-Screen/Elisa was to find out which kind of tablet computer would best fit our target group and the application to be developed. A total number of 30 elderly users, aged from 57 to 91, participated in the test that took place in Germany and Spain. More details of the methodology and results of these tests are published in Burkhard, 2012 (Burkhard and Koch 2012).

SIMPLIT

SIMPLIT is a seal of approval which certifies that a product is comfortable, intuitive and easy to use.[4] To obtain this seal, the product or service must undergo an evaluation process which determines, among other things, the standards of the product and submits it to a usability testing by elderly persons. The SIMPLIT methodology supporting this seal was presented in the 2012 World Conference of the International Society for Gerontechnology (Durá et al. 2012).

The specific application of the SIMPLIT methodology in the SI-Screen/Elisa project consisted of explaining to the user the total number of tasks to be completed during the test (e.g. "go to the interest section" or "make a call"). Once the details were clear, the users were asked to begin with the first task. The time required to perform each of the tasks was recorded. Tasks were performed according to the following procedure:

- Repetition 1: Intuitive performance by a user on their own. If the user performed the task correctly, in a shorter time than the average and without errors, there was no repetition.
- Repetition 2: Support by user's manual. The user repeated the task if it was not performed correctly the first time. The failure criteria were: task did not end successfully, errors were made or the user spent twice the average time. If the user finished the task this second time, the procedure ended.
- Repetition 3: Supported by oral explanations by a technician. The user repeated the task a third time, after an explanation by the technician if the task was not performed properly during the second repetition.
- Repetition 4: Demonstrative training. The task was performed by the technician with the user to confirm that the user had learnt to do the task correctly during the third repetition.

During the validation process, Elisa proved to be very usable. The SIMPLIT methodology gives a combined score of effectiveness and efficiency of use from 0 % (minimum simplicity of use) to 100 % (maximum effectiveness and efficiency of use). The combined tasks analyzed of the second prototype of the Elisa system scored a global value of 99.5 %.

Conjoint analysis

Conjoint analysis (Green and Rao 1971; Green and Srinivasan 1990) is a tool to support decision making as regards the "emotional design" of products and services. This technique determines how people value different features that make up an individual product or service. The development process consists of five main steps:

1. Selection of the product's/service's attributes (i.e. color, material, finishes).
2. Identification of emotional factors (i.e. innovativeness, easiness of use, quality, elegance, robustness).

---

[4] Detailed information about the SIMPLIT seal and methodology is available on the official site http://www.simplit.es/ in English, Spanish and Portuguese.

3. Development of the sample of prototypes to be evaluated on an orthogonal design combining one to one the different attributes.
4. Survey on the users' experiences with a questionnaire containing between twelve and 30 questions designed according to experimental design principles of independence and balance of the attributes.
5. Statistical treatment to support the decision-making in the design process of a product or service. From the statistical treatment, we can obtain the importance of each attribute in relation to on each emotional factor as well as the most and least favorable combination of attributes.

We used this technique to evaluate the second prototype in order to obtain specific design criteria based on the subjective opinions of the elderly people (38 users in Germany and Spain). A total number of eight virtual samples were developed, combining the following attributes: frame color, frame material and finish of stand material.

Task performance and observational protocol
This technique consists of giving the user a set of tasks to be performed and assessing how they perform and perceive those tasks by means of questionnaires and a self-evaluation form.

Task performance was used in the SI-Screen/Elisa project during the validation in a "real" context of the third prototype. We asked the users to take the Elisa tablet home for two weeks. Before the validation we had a training session with the users to explain its purpose and to dispel any doubts regarding the tasks. During the first week, the users had to perform three different tasks per day. At the end of the first week, they had to repeat those tasks to check for improvement. During the second week, users were free to use Elisa whenever they wanted. After each task, the users had to fill in a brief questionnaire and an auto-evaluation template (observational protocol) to record all their impressions, opinions, and general feedback, like the time it took them to perform each of the tasks, the problems they encountered, or their perception of the difficulty.

Field trial
In the field trial technique (Jordan 2000; Poulson et al. 1996) users use the product in "real life" for a predefined period of time. This type of test usually evaluates the use of a product in combination with subjective and objective measures. It is not a recommended technique for the initial design phases.

In the context of the SI-Screen/Elisa project, we used this technique during the validation of the third prototype. To evaluate the use of the product in a real use environment we used a combination of the techniques task performance and observational protocol. After each task, the users had to fill in a brief questionnaire and an auto-evaluation template (observational protocol) to record all impressions, opinions and general feedback such as the length of time each task took, problems encountered, or perceived difficulties. At the end of the field trial, we interviewed the users and carried out a focus group with the participants to share impressions and comments.

Table 2 Example of the application of the Kano model to a TV and the Elisa system

Product	Basic	Performance	Excitement
TV	Color	Flatness	Smart TV
Elisa	Easy to use	Integration "all in one"	Be inspired

Questionnaires (regarding satisfaction)

There are different types of questionnaires (Poulson et al. 1996; Jordan 2000; Poveda et al. 2003b): open, close, ranking, scales, etc. It is necessary to adapt them to the specific area of application; in this case to the needs of elderly people and persons with disabilities.

For the SI-Screen/Elisa project, we used different types of questionnaires depending on the development phase and the information we wanted to obtain from the users. By means of the questionnaires we learned about the users' preferences (different devices or layouts of the GUI), their difficulties in performing the tasks or sociodemographic data (relative to social participation and affinity to technology)

Kano model

The Kano model is a methodology used in product and services design that allows for the classification of the functionalities or requirements of a product or system into three main categories:

- Threshold or basic attributes are basically the features that the product must have in order to meet customer demands. If this attribute is overlooked, the product is simply incomplete.
- Performance attributes are those to which the maxim "the more the better" applies as better performance attributes will improve customer satisfaction. Reversely, weak performance attributes will reduce customer satisfaction. The needs that belong to the performance attribute category are usually those customers would spontaneously name when asked about the attributes they would like to have in a product or service.
- Excitement attributes are for the most part unforeseen by the users but may bring them immense satisfaction as it spurs their imagination. Those attributes might let potential consumers discover needs that they never knew they had.

Table 2 shows an example of the application of the Kano model to a TV as a base of comparison for the application of the Kano model to the Elisa system. We have to keep in mind that excitement attributes can become performance or even basic attributes with time, as was the case for color TV. In the framework of the SI-Screen/Elisa project, the Kano model was used to prioritize the demands of the users as a first step to transforming them into product specifications and functionalities and finally into features to be implemented.

References

Burkhard, M., Koch, M.: Evaluating touchscreen interfaces of tablet computers for elderly people. In: Reiterer, H., Deussen, O. (eds.) Mensch and Computer 2012–Workshopband: interaktiv informiert–allgegenwärtig und allumfassend!?, pp. 53–59. Oldenbourg Verlag, München (2012)

Campos, N.: Metodologías de comercialización y provisión de recursos para la calidad de vida *(Methodologies for trading and allocation of resources for quality of life)* (2010)

Cooper, A.: The origin of personas. http://www.cooper.com/2008/05/15/the_origin_of_personas (2008). Accessed 31 June 2013

Douglas, S.A., Kirkpatrick, A.A.E., MacKenzie, I.S.: Testing pointing device performance and user assessment with the ISO 9241, Part 9 standard. In: Altom, M.W., Williams, M.G. (eds.) Proceedings of the SIGCHI conference on Human factors in computing systems the CHI is the limit CHI 99, 15, pp. 215–222. ACM Press, New York (1999). doi:10.1145/302979.303042

Durá, J.V., Laparra, J., Poveda, R., Marzo, R., Lopez, A., Bollain, C.: SIMPLIT: ensuring technology usability for the elderly. In: Gerontechnology, vol. 11(2). Full paper. http://gerontechnology.info/index.php/journal/article/view/gt.2012.11.02.279.00/1645. (2012)

Economic Commission for Europe of the United Nations (UNECE): Terminology on statistical metadata. In: Conference of European Statisticians Statistical Standards and Studies, No. 53. Geneva (2000)

Green, P.E., Rao, V.R.: Conjoint measurement for quantifying judgmental data. J. Mark. Res. **5**, 103–123 (1971)

Green, P.E., Srinivasan, V.: Conjoint analysis in marketing: new developments with implications for research and practice. J. Mark. Res. **54**, 3–19 (1990)

Grudin, J., Pruitt, J.: Personas, participatory design and product development: an infrastructure for engagement. In: Binder, T., Gregory, J., Wagner, I. (eds.) Proceedings of the Participatory Design Conference, pp. 144–161. Malmöö, Sweeden (2002)

Hasdoğan, G., Evyapan, N., Korkut, F.: Understanding user experience for scenario building: a case in public transportation design. In: Bust, P.D. (ed.) Contemporary Ergonomics, pp. 189–193. Taylor and Francis, London (2006)

Jordan, P.W.: Designing Pleasurable Products. Taylor Francis Ltd, London (2000)

Juriasti, P.: Técnicas de investigación en Ciencias Sociales. Servicio editorial UPV-EHU, Leioa (2003)

Lahuerta, R.: Metodologías para la detección de necesidades y oportunidades de innovación orientada por las personas *(Person Oriented Methodologies to detect needs and innovation opportunitie)*. Book of Proceedings I Foro sobre innovación, economía y calidad de vida, pp. 89–94 (2010). ISBN 978-84-95448-21-7

Nelsen, L.: The ten steps to user personas. HCI VISTAS. Volumen-III, 2007–2008. http://www.hceye.org/HCInsight-Nielsen.htm (2007). Accessed 16 July 2013

Poveda, R., Barberà-Guillem R, Sánchez-Lacuesta, J.: MUSA/IBV. Método para la selección de ayudas técnicas bajo criterios de usabilidad. Instituto de Biomecánica de Valencia. (2003a)

Poveda, R., Barberà-Guillem, R., Cort, JM., Sánchez-Lacuesta, J., Prat, J.: DATUS/IBV ¿Cómo obtener productos con alta usabilidad? Instituto de Biomecánica de Valencia (2003b)

Poulson, D., Ashby, M., Richardson, S.: USERFIT: A Practical Handbook on User-Centred Design for Assistive Technology. ECSC-EC-EAEC, Brussels-Luxembourg (1996)

Pruitt, J.S., Grudin, J.: Personas: Practice and Theory. 2003 ACM 1-58113-728-1 03/0006 5.0 (2003)

Soukoreff, R.W., MacKenzie, I.S.: Towards a standard for pointing device evaluation, perspectives on 27 years of Fitts' law research in HCI. Int. J. Hum. Comput. Stud. **61**(6), 751–789 (2004). doi:10.1016/j.ijhcs.2004.09.001

Statistics Canada: Statistics Canada Quality Guidelines, 3rd edn, p. 7. Oct 1998

Such, M.J.: Metodologías de diseño orientado por las personas (Person Design Oriented Methodologies). Book of Proceedings I Foro sobre innovación, economía y calidad de vida, pp. 107–114 (2010). ISBN 978-84-95448-21-7

Wikipedia Contributors: Heuristic evaluation, Wikipedia, The Free Encyclopedia, 4 July 2013, 15:02, http://en.wikipedia.org/wiki/Heuristic_evaluation (2013). Accessed 5 July 2013

Functions: How We Understood and Realized Functions of Real Importance to Users

Eckehard Fozzy Moritz, Stephan Biel, Martin Burkhard,
Stefanie Erdt, Javier Gámez Payá, Javier Ganzarain,
Michael Koch, Andrea Nutsi and Ute Vidal Cabello

1 Executive Summary

In this chapter, five important functionalities will be discussed that need to be understood and addressed en route to success in person-oriented innovation ventures. Three of these functionalities, communication, be inspired, and information, were identified as core functions for the project SI-Screen/Elisa and were therefore an integral part of this project. However, in this chapter, we also included the discussion of two more functionalities, joy of use and movement motivation. Those were part of Elisa on a more abstract level but they are nonetheless often at least as important for the success of any project as the core functionalities. Moreover, the authors already collected considerable practice experience regarding these functionalities in previous projects that is well worth sharing here.

2 Be Inspired

To improve social interaction, one important approach is to provide people with inspiration they can follow up with action. This function, called "be inspired", is implemented in Elisa as an activity feed that offers information on what is happening in the users' communities (persons) and in their local environment

M. Burkhard · M. Koch · A. Nutsi
Universität der Bundeswehr München, Neubiberg, Germany

S. Biel · J. Ganzarain
Tioman & Partners SL, Barcelona, Spain

U. Vidal Cabello
VIOS Medien GmbH, Gröbenzell, Germany

E. F. Moritz (✉) · S. Erdt · J. Gámez Payá
Innovationsmanufaktur GmbH, Munich, Germany
e-mail: efm@innovationsmanufaktur.com

E. F. Moritz (ed.), *Assistive Technologies for the Interaction of the Elderly,*
Advanced Technologies and Societal Change, DOI: 10.1007/978-3-319-00678-9_5,
© Springer International Publishing Switzerland 2014

(locations) to encourage them to communicate and to participate in (local) activities. In this section, we briefly describe this functionality and the motivation behind it.

The core goal of Elisa is to support the social interaction of its users. Discussing the issue, we identified encouragement as one way to improve social interaction: The users of Elisa are encouraged to communicate with existing contacts and to participate in (local) activities (and thereby meet new people) by Elisa providing awareness of real-life activities of family and friends as well as of local events and offering the means to initiate communication next to the presentation of this information.

In our context, "awareness" refers to an understanding of what activities are happening in the elderlies' social environment affecting their own activities, e.g. what people they know are doing, as well as what events are happening around them.[1] Awareness of others should inspire the elderly person to participate in social activities in their neighborhood and eventually lead to a feeling of belonging and connectedness (Czaja et al. 2006; Goswami et al. 2010).

This support for social interaction was labeled "be inspired" because the functionality provides inspiration for communication and action. In our search for sources of information, we identified so-called Social Network Services (SNS) as the core source for awareness information in addition to standard media like e-mail.

SNS have shown the potential to support their users in building relationships and staying in contact in different domains over the last years. Goswami et al. (2010) conducted a study that investigated the social needs among the elderly and analysed how SNS could support those needs. They found that, similar to younger adults, introducing the elderly to SNS intensifies their bonds with relatives and friends even at large geographical distances. They also discovered that interviewees with basic computer knowledge were familiar with the fundamental concepts of SNS, intro-duced either by family, friends or media. Although the interviewees were generally interested in SNS, they had concerns about the complexity of social networking sites.

In our approach of realizing "be inspired", we decided to unify the activity and content streams from different SNS like Facebook, Google+, Flickr (see Chap-ter "Social Software Integration: How We Integrated Different Interaction Features and Technologies" for an elaboration on the mash-up functionality in Elisa used to connect all these services), and use Elisa to present this information in an innovative way (see Fig. 1).

In the following, we will elaborate further on how and what kind of awareness support was integrated into Elisa for the "be inspired" functionality. For structuring purposes, we will distinguish between the four types of awareness as defined by Gutwin et al. (1996)[2]:

---

[1] See (Dourish and Bellotti 1992) for other interpretations of the awareness concept and its relevance in work group scenarios.

[2] The study from Gutwin et al. (1996) is from the work group support area. However, the types of awareness needed in this area to support interaction also show up in the field of supporting connectedness in communities in general.

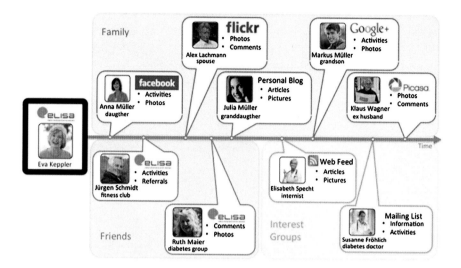

Fig. 1 "Be inspired" as activity stream compiled from different SNS

- Informal awareness
- Social awareness
- Group-structural awareness and
- Workspace awareness.

Informal awareness relates to information on presence, actions and aims of other users. In Elisa, activities of others are perceived via one consistent stream of personal e-mails or status updates of social networking sites, e.g. information on the travels of a grand-child. Moreover, the online status of another person might inspire Elisa users to initiate communication like sending a message or performing a voice or video call (Figs. 2 and 3).

Another type of activity stream conveys happenings in the near environment and who is participating in these events. This function is located in the activities section of Elisa, which shows activities according to the user's interests. An example would be an Elisa user who is interested in photography and gets information about a photography workshop he can participate in. In the activities section in the Elisa user interface, the elderly person may join an event or invite contacts. Therefore, the user is inspired about happenings in the neighborhood, resulting in social activities.

The second awareness type is social awareness, which is defined as information on interests, emotional states and the attention of other users—aspects typically noticed in a personal conversation. The friends section of Elisa contains the contacts' profiles which include contact information, interests and hobbies. This makes it easier for the user to get in contact with people he or she already knows, but also supports the formation of new relationships with people sharing the same interests.

Fig. 2 Loneliness and
isolation

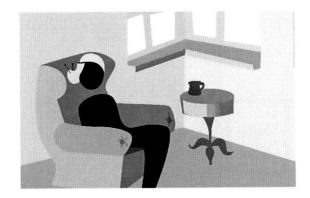

Fig. 3 New forms of
communication and contact

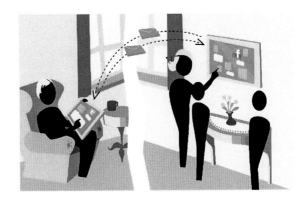

Therefore, the users might be inspired to strengthen and enlarge their personal
networks. Similar to the actions of other users, the emotional state might also be
included in emails or status messages. Furthermore, the emotional state and the
attention can be conveyed in a voice or video call. This inspires a personal contact
with relatives or friends who cannot be met in person, for example due to a large
geographical distance.

Group-structural awareness means general information about a group and its
members, for example their roles, responsibilities, statuses and positions. In Elisa,
the group-structural awareness is realized via an address book listing all contacts
of a user. This address book links to the personal profile view, which also contains
the group, which can be either family or friend. The address book might inspire the
Elisa user to look at the profile of a person he has not contacted recently, see the
updates of this person, and eventually write or call. Consequently, the address
book might foster social interaction and strengthen the personal network.

Workspace awareness is not as easy to find in the Elisa setup since Elisa is
intended for a target group that is largely retired. An example for this type of
awareness would be two people being aware of mutual changes to the same
document. If not collaboratively working on documents, Elisa users can at least
access articles on different topics which are of interest to them. Notifications on

what articles and what additional information on the articles exists therefore can be seen as some kind of workspace awareness. This kind of awareness information is presented in the interests section of the Elisa application. The aim is to provide the latest information and trends, for example new trends in chess that the user might apply in the next meeting of the chess club. The purpose of such related information is to present advice on further reading, events and helpful social contacts. For example, related information of a Diabetes article would propose Diabetes self-help groups near the current reading location. Therefore, the inspiration provided by articles and related content in the interests section of Elisa could also increase social interaction and lead to real-life meetings.

Summing up, the "be inspired" functionality pervades the whole Elisa application. Due to a raised awareness about family, friends and social activities, the elderly user is inspired to increase his or her social activity, to strengthen existing ties and to establish new relationships. The "be inspired" functionality and its joyful implementation and visualization are also key to the "joy of use" metafunctionality described in Sect. 5.

3 Communication

Communication is essential for all human beings. With communication a person can announce her/his needs and interact socially. A lack of communication is therefore one of the main reasons for loneliness which indeed is a serious problem among elderly people. In fact, a growing number of elderly people is isolated, does not have visitors from one week to another, and rarely speaks to other people.

To avoid deterioration of social and familial relationships, elderly people must be encouraged to communicate.

During our requirements' analysis for Elisa, we gained a lot of insights into how the elderly communicate. They want to feel that real contact has been made with someone, that a level of intimacy has been reached, and that they have put something of themselves into the act, or indeed the art, of communication. This is reflected in our test persons' wish to dedicate time to creating thoughtful and reflective communication.

We also gained a lot of insight into which kind of technical devices elderly people are using to communicate with others. In this regard, the most important barrier to their using a computer is actually a perceived lack of benefit. This means that either the technology does not meet their needs, or they do not understand the technology sufficiently to appreciate its benefits. While research participants stated face-to-face contact as their preferred option, they also regarded new technologies as useful and acceptable alternatives and opportunities. The main perceived benefit of those new technologies was their use as an extension of face-to-face communication and as a means of bringing the world into their homes thus providing more contact and stimulation. As an example, the benefits for non-tech-savvy users of "almost being there", that is, of "seeing" the family even though they were in

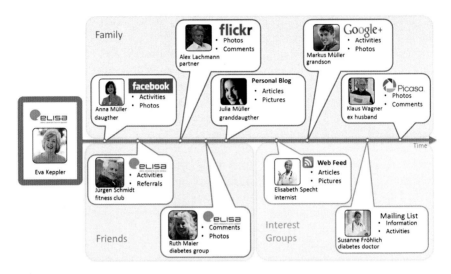

Fig. 4 Social interaction of Eva Keppler with her family and friends as well the latest activities from her interest groups

Australia, were considered priceless. In fact, communicating with the family and breaching increasing distances to remain in contact with loved ones is a great incentive for the elderly to adopt change and use new technologies.

To generate a real benefit, Elisa's further focus lay on creating a joyful and learnable graphical user interface that is capable of adapting to different kinds of users and their diverse experience levels.

As consequence of all of the above, the centre of Elisa's communication functionality is the people and their interaction by written text, voice or video communication. On the one hand, an individual can communicate with another person (one-to-one) by talking on the phone, writing an e-mail or (instant) messages or commenting on provided content (articles, activities, photos etc.). On the other hand, individuals can communicate with several other persons (many-to-many) by having a telephone or video call or participating in textual chats. Figures 4, 5 and 6 show typical examples of such social interaction flows.

The approach developed for Elisa consists of implicit communication and context-aware information instead of the creation of just another e-mail client. Sharing information (see Fig. 7) and inviting other people to join in conversations or activities (see Fig. 8) are some of the main aspects that people will be able to do with Elisa.

However, for usability's sake, this should be done without copying information from a web browser to an e-mail client. By just adding contacts to the information page the conversation can start right away, even if the personal contacts are not members of Elisa. The same approach can also be used for other functionalities: If an elderly person adds friends to a discovered activity, the system automatically sends an invitation to the friend's e-mail address (see Fig. 9).

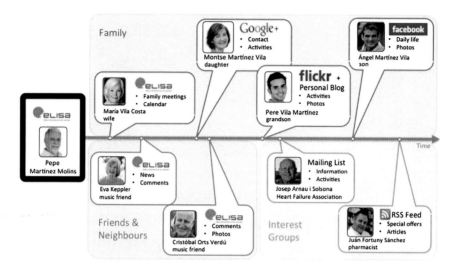

Fig. 5 Social interaction of Pepe Martínez Molins with his family and friends as well as the latest activities of his interest group and his pharmacist

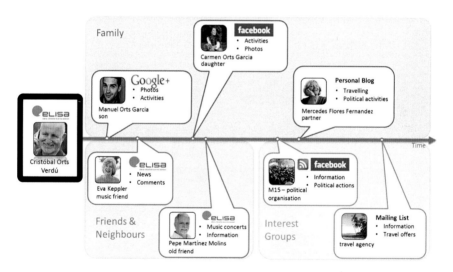

Fig. 6 Social interaction of Christobal Orts Verdú with his family and friends as well as the latest activities of his political interest group and his travel agency

All of the above has, however, only been a first glimpse into the research on communication and the way we took its results into account. Further information will be given in other chapters or—even better—as soon as you use Elisa yourself.

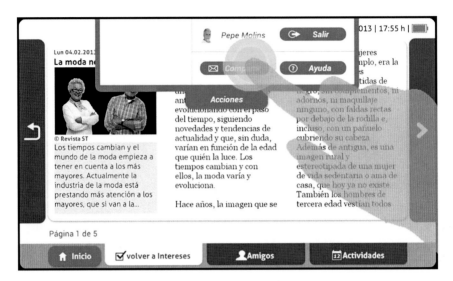

Fig. 7 Sharing information of interest with a contact

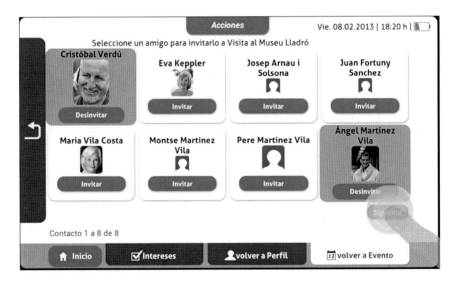

Fig. 8 Inviting friends to join an activity

4 Information

At the beginning of the SI-Screen/Elisa project, we executed a requirements'
analysis. We learned that the functionality most used by elderly internet users is
information, followed by sending and receiving e-mails. Therefore, it seemed self-

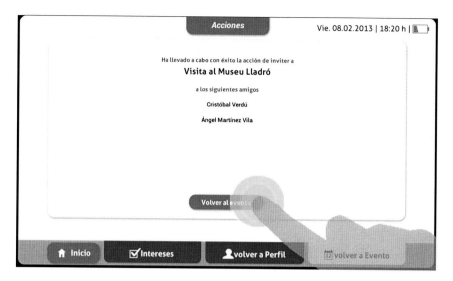

Fig. 9 Getting system feedback about the invitation sent

evident that "information" should be implemented as one of the core function-alities. But during the following discussions we discovered that the functionality "information" is closely interconnected with "be inspired" (see Sect. 2), like two sides of one coin: "Be inspired" offers information users are interested in advance (with the aim to encourage them to communicate and participate in activities). "Information" means that users have to become active themselves to look for this information. Keeping in mind that Elisa wants to especially address users with little or even no experience, we decided to focus on the "be inspired" functionality during the testing of the prototype in the living environment, because on the one hand, in our experience "information", that is, using searching machines, requires a more advanced user and on the other hand, the "be inspired" functionality seemed to be more innovative. Therefore, the utilization of the internet as source of information is described mainly in Sect. 2 "Be inspired".

In this chapter, we will address more general aspects of information, such as the general information behavior of elderly people, their problems dealing with the internet as a source of information, the topics they are interested in and the importance of trusted local offers and information adapted to their interests.

During the analysis phase we asked the online poll participants and the focus groups in Valencia, Barcelona and Munich where they looked for information to plan their daily activities, their leisure time, their travels etc. In both countries, the internet is the third most popular source of information, after newspapers and personal recommendations, followed by magazines and the radio (there are, however, some differences in the range between Germany and Spain, e.g. in Spain, personal recommendations are the most important source of information and in Germany, magazines are more used than in Spain, see Table 1). Even some of the

Table 1 How do you get information on leisure activities in your environment?

(Figures in %)	Germany	Spain
Newspapers	25	24
Talking with friends/personal recommendations	22	25
Internet	18	20
Magazines	13	9
Radio	12	15
Magazines of pharmacies	6	5

(*Source* project online survey conducted in Spain and Germany in 2010)

Social Animal and Shy Guy types with no PC or internet connection of their own mentioned that they receive web-based information from family members or friends.

Generally, the participants considered an almost unlimited access to information and knowledge one of the great advantages of the internet. At the same time, however, they complained strongly that they often feel deluged with information and cannot evaluate its quality. To give an example: A search of information concerning "prevention of hypertension" resulted in about 283.000 hits (Google, July 2013). To find the "good" websites with qualified information and local offers and activities among them is a great problem not only for elderly people.

Elisa was expected to act as a "supervisory authority" for trusted information and reliable sources and as "filter" for undesirable information—especially "useless" information and advertisements. It was important to not only find technical solutions for implementing different information streams in the interest, friends and activity sections of Elisa but also to ensure the quality of the selected information channels and their fitting to the interests of the users. As there is an enormous and constantly growing amount of websites and data in the internet, this will be an ongoing task of a future Elisa commercialization.

Despite the fact that interests depend on a person rather than their age, we still found topics that a great part of people over 50 years are interested in. In the interest section we summarized them in the following categories: "society" (e.g. politics, voluntary engagement), "culture" (e.g. history, tradition), "travelling" (e.g. travel destinations, hotels), "health & wellbeing" (e.g. disease treatments, health tips) and "living & care" (new residential arrangements, care offers). In the activity section the categories are: "culture" (e.g. concerts, theater), "health & fitness" (e.g. Nordic walking, biking), "trips & guided tours" (e.g. excursions, museums), "workshops & classes" (e.g. languages, painting), "my city" (e.g. festivities, fairs). In order to avoid receiving undesirable information, every user can configure Elisa to his or her interests with just a few clicks (see Figs. 10 and 11): If a category is deselected, Elisa does not present articles or activities on this topic.

Once again, we have to remember the core aim of Elisa: to enable elderly people to communicate easily with others and help them to find and participate in

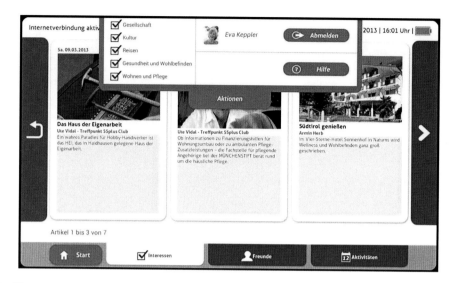

Fig. 10 Categories in the interest section to be selected or deselected

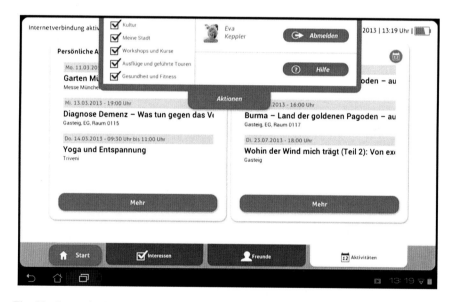

Fig. 11 Categories in the activity section to be selected or deselected

local activities, health and wellbeing offers. To motivate Elisa users to participate in activities and invite friends to take part as well, it was important to focus on information about local activities and offers. Why local? First of all, a great part of the daily (leisure) activities takes place in the near environment of people. Nobody likes travelling two hours every week just to take part in an English conversation class of 45 min! Information on local events and offers thus makes it easier for an Elisa user to take part at short notice, e.g. to join the Nordic walking group in the nearby park in the afternoon and invite a friend to this event.

Summing up, the quality of the information or better, the usefulness of the content presented in the sections "interests", "friends" and "activities" is essential to achieving Elisa's aim of increasing the amount of social activity of the elderly as described in the "be inspired" functionality and the "joy of use" (see Sects. 2 and 5, respectively).

5 Joy of Use

Maximized use value ... this demand is almost omnipresent in this book, and rightfully so. The question we like to address now is, apart from practical and technical functions, in how far do emotional factors contribute to this use value of a product? And also, which ones, and how do innovators take care of them?

To be sure, nice designs, fanciful fashioning and smart positioning are certainly factors that contribute to the success of a product: Industrial designers and marketing agents are often enough not only more in number but also better paid than the good old engineer, especially in lifestyle companies. Our argument in the following will be that a concentration on joy of use is not only gravely neglected in comparison to the above mentioned emotional functionalities, but that it is extremely important to catalyze the realization of other functionalities and thus maximize the actual use of a product (and hence help perform the practical functionalities at all).

The story of our first practical encounter with this phenomenon will easily illustrate what we mean by this argument. A task we had embarked on 5 years ago was to develop an idea and knowledge platform for the German Ski Association to which as many of those involved in the success of the national team in alpine skiing as possible should contribute and integrate their knowledge and expertise. Obviously, the success of a knowledge platform depends on the amount of knowledge existing on the platform: It will only become the habitual tool of choice if more than a critical mass of those concerned will be using it. But how do you make trainers, waxers, and overly busy scientists use this platform, especially since at the beginning a still virgin data basis is still of little use, and putting in new data is perceived by many to be more work than they may ever get out of it.

The secret remedy we resorted to was to develop a platform that embodied "joy of use". Much more than just being user-friendly or easy to use, this meant that the use itself is supposed to be joy, regardless of the practically intended use. As the idea to optimize the platform towards more joy of use even created a sort of "joy of development", quite a number of features were created with just that objective in mind. Among these were

- lists of songs preferred by many users of the platform
- a continuous stream of stimulating and/or funny videos
- unconventional access options to the platform, and to the integration of knowledge (e.g. the "no idea where this belongs to, but I need to tell you" but-ton)
- the opportunity to phone, write emails and SMS to the platform
- humorous discussions in the blog.

The effect was just as intended: We got more users to use the platform more often for more purposes: The platform itself hence became much more useful, and a role model for knowledge support in German top sports until today. There is much knowledge represented and it constantly increases, and there are often effects of serendipity even today: You find interesting things that you were not really looking for, and are stimulated for novel action.

When designing Elisa, we tried to keep these ideas in mind. Elisa should not only provide functions to communicate and to access information in an easy to use way, but also be joyful to use.

One aspect of joy of use was to provide personal user experiences and to surprise the user (see Sect. 5.1 and (Reeps 2004)). This is covered in Elisa by focusing on people instead of content. We do not provide simple content feeds in Elisa, but information about people the user knows or information that is connected to people she or he might want to know. This provides a personal user experience and some (positive) surprise from time to time. When going through the list of functions in the rest of this chapter, the function "be inspired" is of key importance.

The other aspect of joy of use we tried to address in the concept is the flow aspect (see Sect. 5.1). Flow is achieved when the application provides adequate challenges and a control of the situation. In the Elisa concept we tried to contribute to this by dynamically adapting the available functions in the user interface to the level of experience of the user. In the beginning, a user gets just a few options, but the more experienced he or she gets with the user interface the more options are provided.

5.1 Scientific Excursion

With "joy of use" we introduced an expression that is apparently self-explanatory on the one hand, but invites of a large variety of interpretations and definitions on the other. In the literature we can even find something as complicated as: "Joy of use is the pleasurable experience of the quality of interaction and the opportunities, which for a certain user in a certain context mean a mostly unobtrusive outstanding performance and a motivated use of the software according to the objectives and interests of a user due to an esthetically ambitious design" (Hatscher 2001).

While the definition itself neither shows any joy of use for designers nor for most of the readers, we like to approach an understanding of this important topic by firstly deconstructing it: Whereas the term "use" is seemingly very clear, the component "joy" is more demanding to understand, describe, and make accessible to developers. Not having found a really useful definition of "joy" itself, we have decided to approximate it from three sides, all fully or partly constituents of joy: fun, flow, and pleasure.

- **Fun** is an emotional state related to action, pleasure and disconnection. There is no need to concentrate on the action, because "you know anytime and without reflecting what is the right thing to do." (Rheinberg 1997, p. 143; whole citation Moritz and Steffen 2003). According to early experimentations by Moritz, fun may be felt due to the experience of self-assertion, appreciation, self-competence, an experience of positive esthetics or physiologic feelings, an unexpected positive surprise, the successful mastering of a challenge, or creative aspects of work.
- **Flow** is a much better defined concept especially well received in many aspects of sports and leisure. It originates from Csikszentmihalyi (1985) and means the complete immersion in an action without need for any reflection.
- **Pleasure**, finally, has been distinguished from fun by Blythe and Hassenzahl (2003) as being related to absorption, whereas fun is more related to distraction. Even though we do not completely agree, this distinction offers yet more relevant aspects to reflect upon.

More helpful is the deconstruction of pleasure into different categories, and again different hierarchies, leading to the pleasure hierarchy by Holt and Lock (2008) shown in Fig. 12, which defines numerous instances of what really constitutes pleasure.

To complement the reflections on pleasure, one needs to distinguish between the pleasure while anticipating an event, while experiencing it, and even after it, especially if it was successful or otherwise memorably pleasurable. Finally, similar to fun, what is regarded as pleasure does not only depend on an activity itself but also on different dimensions of its context and, most difficult to master, on the personality, the "pleasure type".

Summarizing all of these considerations, on the one hand it becomes clear that joy of use is certainly a much more complex phenomenon than we originally may have thought. On the other hand, they also helped us to structure joy better (Fig. 13), and derive a number of concrete sub-functionalities that are more easily accessible to analysis and development than the ambiguous "joy of use".

On the basis of this model it quickly becomes clear that any development work intended to provide a basis for joy of use must start with an understanding of what "joy types" the intended users are.

There is certainly much more general research to be done, but especially if you develop for a user group with little overlap to your own psychological and intellectual set-up it is highly likely that for them "joy of use" may mean

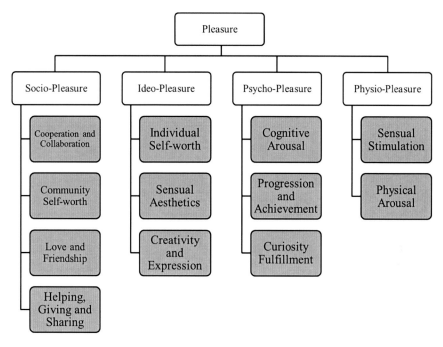

Fig. 12 Pleasure hierarchy by Holt and Lock (2008)

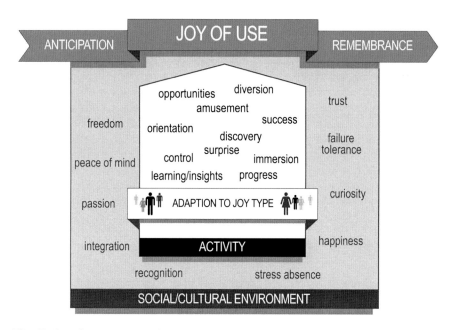

Fig. 13 Joy of use—a system view

something very different from your own interpretation (unfortunately, this fact is often neglected by developers…).

On that basis, product developers should concentrate their efforts on providing joyful experiences in the activity performed with the product in question. (Likely, developers cannot much influence the environment, but they should nonetheless be aware of its importance and possibly even urge those who do have some influence to help foster a respective environment, e.g. regarding trust, failure tolerance, and stress reduction). More specifically, developers should provide the basis for:

- Surprise: Users will experience (positive) things they did not expect.
- Progress: Users will (have the impression to) advance to what they intended.
- Immersion: Users will not need to, even forget to, think about and reflect upon what they are doing.
- Orientation: Users will at any time know exactly what to do in order to progress.
- Control: Users will always (have the feeling to) be in charge about what happens.
- Learning/insights: Users will experience the feeling of having acquired new knowledge or new conceptions.
- Amusement: Users will be inspired to smile, even laugh.
- Discovery: Users will get to know things of their interest that they were not looking for.
- Opportunities: Users will always have choices regarding how they use the product.
- Diversion: Users will be entertained and will experience a playful mindset.
- Success: Users will at least reach their intended goals.

When looking at the list of fun, flow and pleasure (see above) one also might think of a relation to games which are also applications that have to provide joy because they often do not have a practical use. Thus, it is not surprising, that many of the concepts discussed above can be found in games. Detecting successful concepts in games, and using them in other domains has thus become quite popular only recently under the term "gamification" (Deterding et al. 2011).

Of course it is all but easy to perform all of these functions and hence provide joy of use. But for almost all products intended for users directly, the effort will definitely pay off. And, to conclude, the two best ways to achieve this are empathy with the users and "joy of work" in your own development activities.

6 Movement Motivation

In this section we will address an issue that has been relevant only at the fringes of this project, but is of big importance to the success of many, especially health-related, AAL projects.

What we found out, partly in this but especially in other projects, actually sounds quite commonplace: Activities theoretically beneficial to preventive health promotion will in practice only have an effect if they are in fact carried out. But the less immediate a health problem appears to people, e.g. by pains or limitations in movement, the less likely it is that they will engage in preventive activities. In short, health promotion is in general an important action motivator for people, but usually not one that engenders concrete activity.

All of this has one important consequence: An increase of the attractiveness of constitutional activities is needed to boost the effect of health promotion. In the following, we will therefore summarize theoretical knowledge and practical experiences regarding the increase of attractiveness of one of the most important preventive activities: physical movement. We will end with a few insights into how this can and did influence our work in AAL projects in general and SI-Screen/ Elisa in particular.

At the very beginning of the project, our target group was polled regarding their motivation to exercise. Almost 400 people in Germany and Spain filled in the questionnaire online or in a personal interview, at which moment more than 200 people were over 40 years old.

As a result of the poll and other preliminary studies, we realized the poster "fight the inner demon" (see Fig. 14). This poster is a first graphical approach to understand the complex issue of movement motivations and barriers for the elderly and their importance for the innovation process.

From our perspective, this has become necessary as the classic, centuries-old perception of health as the absence of sickness propagated by medical science is outdated. Rather, following the WHO's definition, health has to be interpreted as a state of physical, mental, and social well-being. The most promising approach to general well-being is a fair amount of sports or exercise combined with healthy nourishment.

Intellectually, most people know that. However, there is quite a big discrepancy between the percentage of people who plan to exercise more and those who actually do so. This is perfectly illustrated by the might of everyone's weaker self, their "inner demon". Especially among the elderly, the percentage of active people declines appreciably. Therefore, it is even more important to identify how this target group's movement motivation develops and how exercise at that age can be stimulated systematically.

Apart from physicians' advice to exercise more, the goal has to be to stimulate the intrinsic motivation to do sports in order to develop more directed strategies to conquer one's "inner demon". The newly designed poster therefore correlates attitudes towards health with barriers (the weaker self) and motivators (defeating that inner demon). As an extension of the insights into motivation in the last chapter, the best agers typically needing more exercise are divided into three groups: the Couch Potatoes, the Postponers and the Sanitary Theorists.

The descriptions in Table 2 are based on the study mentioned above.

Apart from catering to motivators, new solutions also have to integrate their individual approach to health promotion into the best agers' living environments in

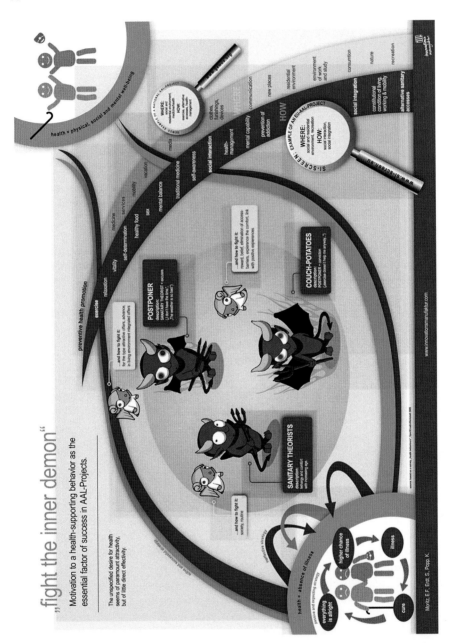

Fig. 14 Poster "fight the inner demon"

Table 2 Short description of the types of movement motivation

Qualities of couch potatoes	Possibilities to defeat their weaker self:
They • do no more than what is absolutely necessary • neglect their health/perceive it as sufficient • have little personal responsibility	• rewards • persuasion • elimination of high entry thresholds • give a better understanding of well-being • link to positive experiences
Qualities of postponers	Possibilities to defeat their weaker self:
They • often decide to do something for their health but never become active • find countless excuses why sport is not possible at a given moment • are Bon Vivants, feel fit and healthy • have almost no prevention • have a tendency to slide into a risk group	• type-related attractive offers • give a better understanding of progress • offers integrated into their living environment
Qualities of sanitary theorists	Possibilities to defeat their weaker self:
They • think they confidently handle their health • become increasingly lethargic and comfortable in old age • have theoretically no problems to live healthily • put independence, family and reputation at the center • are open towards health technology and auto-diagnosis	• connect activities to social contacts • daily routines

order to be successful. One innovative solution from another AAL project that might in future even become connected to Elisa is the movement/exercise chair "Gewos" (from German "Gesund wohnen mit Stil", living healthily in style). It is a normal arm chair that can easily and swiftly be transformed into a fitness machine connected to the TV. It thus provides a low-threshold possibility for exercise that is adapted to the elderlies' living environment as well as their general state of fitness and, last but not least, their needs and wants.

SI-Screen/Elisa as well ties in with a basic need; in this case social interaction. SI-Screen/Elisa has researched how social interaction in this age group can be simplified and how offers beneficial to their health can be connected to the best agers' communication patterns.

References

Blythe, M., Hassenzahl, M.: The semantics of fun: differentiating enjoyable experiences. In: Blythe, M.A., Overbeeke, K., Monk, A.F., Wright, P.C. (eds.) Funology: From Usability to Enjoyment, pp. 91–100. Kluwer Academic Publishers, Dordrecht (2003)

Csikszentmihalyi, M.: Das Flow-Erlebnis. Klett-Cotta, Stuttgart (1985)

Czaja, S.J.S., et al.: Factors predicting the use of technology: findings from the Center for Research and Education on Aging and Technology Enhancement (CREATE). Psychol. Aging **21**(2), 333–352 (2006)

Deterding, S., Khaled, R., Nacke, L., Dixon, D.: Gamification: toward a definition. In: Proceedings Workshop on Gamification at the ACM International Conference on Human Factors in Computing Systems (CHI), (2011)

Dourish, P., Bellotti, V.: Awareness and coordination in shared workspaces. In: Proceedings of the 1992 ACM Conference on Computer-Supported Cooperative Work - CSCW '92, pp. 107–114. ACM Press, New York (1992)

Goswami, S., et al.: Using online social networking to enhance social connectedness and social support for the elderly. In: Proceedings of the International Conference on Information Systems (ICIS), pp. 107–132. Saint Louis, MO, USA (2010)

Gutwin, C., Greenberg, S., Roseman, M.: Workspace awareness in real-time distributed groupware: framework, widgets, and evaluation. In: People and Computers (1996)

Hatscher, M.: Joy of use – determinanten der Freude bei der software-nutzung. In: Oberquelle, H., Oppermann, R., Krause, J. (Hrsg.) Mensch und Computer 2001: 1. Fachübergreifende Konferenz, pp. 343–352. Teubner BG, Stuttgart (2001)

Holt, J., Lock, S.: Understanding and deconstructing pleasure: a hierarchical approach, CHI 2008. April 5–10 (2008)

Moritz, E.F., Steffen, J.: Test For Fun – ein Konzept für einen nutzerorientierten Sportgerätetest. In: Roemer, K., Edelmann-Nusser, J., Witte, K., Moritz, E.F. (Hrsg.) Sporttechnologie zwischen Theorie und Praxis. Shaker Verlag, Aachen (2003)

Rheinberg, F.: Motivation. Kohlhammer, Stuttgart (1997)

Reeps, I.E.: State-of-the-Art Analyse – Usability, Design und Joy of Use. Retrieved from http://hci.uni-konstanz.de/downloads/STAR_Reeps.pdf (2004). Accessed 5 Aug 2013

Design: How We Attempted to Attract Users in Optics, Haptics, and Ease of Utilization

Steffen Ganz, Hannes Pasqualini, Isacco Chiaf, Jan Kliewer
and Martin Burkhard

1 Hardware Design

1.1 Executive Summary

In this section, we will describe in detail how we created the different prototypes that were presented to the test persons during various stages of the Elisa development process.

1.2 Main Results

At the end of the project SI-Screen/Elisa, a physical prototype with a leather frame, an additional frame and the Elisa software was created. Its origin story is described in this section.

1.3 Storyline

Concept phase

As we commenced the project the general task was clear: We wanted to provide a "window to the digital world" to allow elderly people to benefit from the achievements of today's technology in terms of new ways of communication and

S. Ganz (✉)
Porsche Design Studio, Zell am See, Austria
e-mail: s.ganz@porsche-design.at

H. Pasqualini · I. Chiaf · J. Kliewer
Helios, Bolzano, Italy
e-mail: hpasqualini@helios.bz

M. Burkhard
Universität der Bundeswehr München, Neubiberg, Germany

E. F. Moritz (ed.), *Assistive Technologies for the Interaction of the Elderly*,
Advanced Technologies and Societal Change, DOI: 10.1007/978-3-319-00678-9_6,
© Springer International Publishing Switzerland 2014

being part of the various social digital networks out there. Initially, the different partners did not have a common vision about what kind of product would result from the upcoming three years of work. So, we discussed the direction of the main concept together in several workshops to figure out the basic product idea.

For some partners Elisa was some kind of software that realizes all the elderly people's wishes and needs with a unique user interface that combines the different communication services like video telephony, organizing contacts and providing simple access to the different social networks. When thinking of that kind of tool, everything is still only an issue on the software side. So, some sort of Elisa-application running on an existing tablet PC, for example, seems to be enough.

But other partners raised the justified question: How do we bring the elderly to use any application when they do not even have the proper technical devices at home?

Actually, the first obstacles for our target group are to be found much earlier. First, if one wants to catch elderly people's attention, something tangible is needed. Since we know that the elderly to quite some degree are rather uneasy around technical devices, they need a device which is specifically designed for their needs, regarding safety, quality, durability, ease of use, flexibility, the user interface and the functions and mobility of the device.

Since SI-Screen/Elisa as a whole was—as mentioned previously—set up as a Holistic Innovation venture, the partners developed the idea to combine a new user interface with hardware specifically designed for the elderly.

For creating those visions designers have the right skills and tools and are able to make them visible. Visualizations and drawings inspire the group and project a common idea in the minds of all partners. In the following month we were thinking of concepts which can fulfil all the requests and incorporate the demanded functions. Moreover, we analyzed the current products on the market regarding their adaptability to the elderly people's needs.

Design descriptions

The first outstanding design element of the new Elisa product design is the surrounding leather-covered frame. Our main intention for the design was to reduce the elderlies' fear of technical systems and devices. Therefore, we designed this frame in such a way that it allows people to grasp Elisa from every side without touching the sensitive display area. It also serves as a protection for the device in case of a fall (Figs. 1, 2 and 3).

Our Elisa product focuses on aspects like ease of use, comfort and security instead of the emphasis on making tablet PCs as thin and light as possible or using high-tech materials, which is the current approach of the tablet-manufacturers on the market. The "thinness" of technical products stands for state of the art technology—this is a trend Elisa doesn't have to follow, our focus is different. Accordingly, we not only covered the surrounding of the glass with leather and employed a combination of authentic materials used for making furniture like glass, aluminum or leather to replace or cover plastic parts. These authentic materials, comfortable for the user, promote the uniqueness of the prototype, and

Fig. 1 Elisa concept
visualization

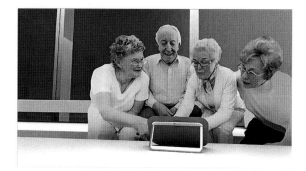

Fig. 2 Elisa product with an
additional bag and a stand

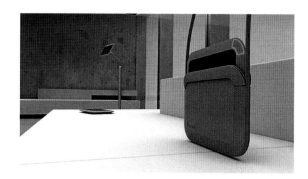

Fig. 3 Elisa tablet device—
cushioned frame with grip
zone

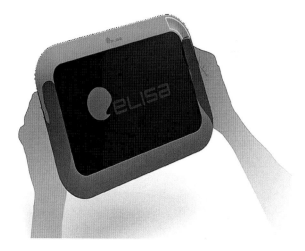

raise the level of customer appreciation. Assuming that our target group will hold
the device for a long time, we have covered the whole back part of Elisa with
leather to increase durability.

Apart from the soft framing for the grip zone, we also realized a softly shaped
back part. In addition, we elaborated a solid stand (Fig. 4), easily accessible and

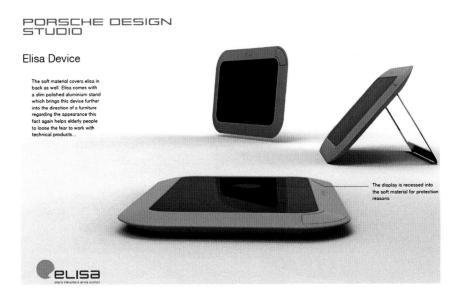

PORSCHE DESIGN
STUDIO

Elisa Device

The soft material covers elisa in
back as well. Elisa comes with
a slim polished aluminium stand
which brings this device further
into the direction of a furniture
regarding the appearance this
fact again helps elderly people
to loose the fear to work with
technical products...

The display is recessed into
the soft material for protection
reasons

ⒺLISƎ
elderly interaction & service assistant

Fig. 4 Elisa design description front

providing the perfect angle for a safe two-hand-operation for interacting with the Elisa UI. Having safety but also portability in mind, a rubber handle (Fig. 5) was attached to the back to allow for safe transport. All in all, the combination of the leather-covering of the device together with authentic materials, the sturdy stand and the handle bar should convey the feeling that damaging sensitive and precious technology is not possible.

Prototypes

The actual product realization with regard to the hardware design commenced with the development of different prototypes. Three prototype phases were scheduled within the period of time for the project; each of the phases was followed by an iteration and refinement phase (Figs. 6, 7 and 8).

The first prototype was planned for nine months after the project start. At that time, we wanted to validate and firstly test the overall Elisa concept and our product vision together with a prototype of the Elisa UI (user interface). For examining the holistic design concept of Elisa, we developed realistic computer aided visualizations of the expected use case scenarios based on a target group use case story. These use case scenarios, internally called Ambient Settings (AS), are intended to give our test persons an overview of the benefits the device should provide. We expected valuable information from this survey not only regarding the concept itself, but also with respect to the perception of the product in terms of appearance, functionality and handling aspects. The mockup of the Elisa UI prototype consisted of a common android tablet PC (which was then available on the market) with our Elisa software installed. Thus this prototype was not a design model which could have represented our picture of the Elisa product by means of

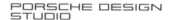

Elisa Device

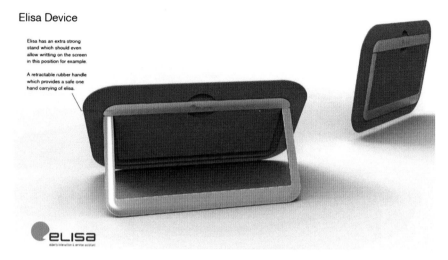

Elisa has an extra strong
stand which should even
allow writting on the screen
in this position for example.

A retractable rubber handle
which provides a safe one
hand carrying of elisa.

Fig. 5 Elisa design description back

Fig. 6 Elisa design model
front

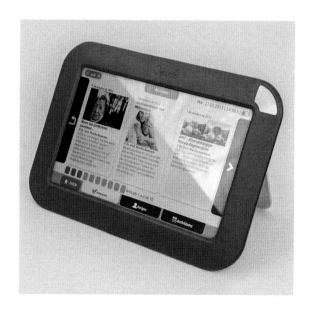

realizing the true product appearance of Elisa as shown in the design description
and renderings on the prior pages.

The second prototype (scheduled three months after the first one) was intended
to be the first physical prototype representative for our design proposal in shape
and dimensions. This mockup was mainly made in the model shop of the Porsche

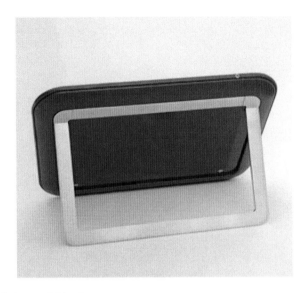

Fig. 7 Elisa design model back

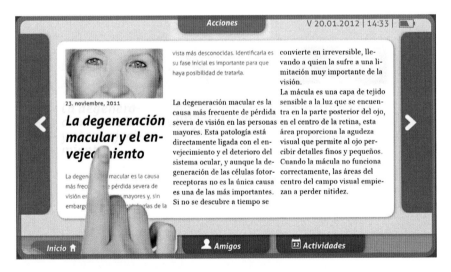

Fig. 8 Natural interaction with the Elisa user interface

Design Studio. After the first refinement phase, we had incorporated all the insights and feedback from the testing and validation results. We had also implemented these adjustments into the 3D data of the Elisa device. At this point, we were able to start building one physical mockup by milling the Elisa shape out of a special modeling foam. Into this first housing, we inserted the technical components of one of our android tablets with the Elisa software. With this mockup, we followed the approach to create an operating mockup on which we can test several things like the positions of the buttons, the operation of the stand and the refined functions of the Elisa UI. After the testing of this prototype the second iteration phase took place.

Realization options

For the development and manufacturing of this prototype there are basically two possibilities. Since no manufacturer and no engineering company took part in this project, we had to think about the right steps to be taken to prepare everything for a possible production of Elisa ourselves.

- Option 1: Development as an original equipment manufacturer (OEM) of a tablet based on our industrial design. An OEM partner manufactures products or components that are purchased by a company and distributed under that purchasing company's brand name.
- Option 2: Production through a contract manufacturer electronic manufacturing services (EMS). Usage of the android tablet kits plus production of the housing, including assembly, packaging, etc.

We considered the second option to be more realistic, because the production volume (especially for the first stage) will probably be low (<100.000 units). In this case, it will be difficult to find a manufacturer. Based on a certain android tablet PC platform which fits our needs, there are numerous EMS which were considered.

Of course, the housing must be developed (like injection of mold parts, fixation of internal technical components etc.). In addition, the integration of the product has to be processed. Some EMS can do it internally, because they have in-house development teams, others do not. We had to consider the question whether it made sense to involve as a third party, an engineering agency for this further development which, however was not part of this project. On the one hand, the internal team of a manufacturer usually has the advantage of lower initial costs and the design transfer is seamless. However, the customer (in this case, us) has only limited control over the costs. Furthermore, the customer usually does not have control over the complete documentation and rights of the design because some engineering takes place within the manufacturer's workplace. An external development agency on the other hand works for the interests of its customer without exception, with fully documented design, which would give us the opportunity to keep a clear picture of the production costs. Therefore, the costs are usually lower in a long-term view, and the production can be shifted to another manufacturer at a certain point if necessary.

We would thus pledge to cooperate with an engineering agency in the future to make sure that all developments and ideas remain in the hands of the consortium and our acquired knowledge would not be used in a non-appropriate manner. To be involved in the process over a longer period of time during the development would have diverse advantages, especially for the quality management of the product. In any case, we had to find manufacturers/suppliers of android tablet PC kits which can be built into our Elisa hardware design in parallel to the ongoing second refinement phase.

After finishing the second refinement phase and before starting with the development of the third prototype (scheduled around nine months after the second prototype), we needed to have a so-called "design freeze" which means that we had to agree on the specifications of the industrial design. After that, shape, color, surface finishes, parts and materials are fixed. After the design freeze we could build the third prototype, the design model representing the outer product form identical to the later production model. The surfaces, fonts, colours and moving parts were reproduced exactly. The design model is therefore suitable for photos or brochure presentations at trade fairs and in the end serves as a reference and documentation for quality and exactness of the appearance for the manufacturer at a later stage. The finished product design can be provided for further processing (mainly for construction) with the main dimensions. In our case, the detailing by design engineers will be necessary to create a technical drawing for the batch production.

In the end, the design model always serves as a reference and documentation for quality and exactness of the appearance in the final months of the project.

2 User Interface Design

2.1 Executive Summary

The work on the graphical user interface (GUI) and user experience for the Elisa system was mainly focused on the creation of a new, touch-oriented metaphor for the interface, which could be easier to understand and more straightforward to use for the elderly people.

2.2 Main Results

By abandoning the traditional WIMP (windows, icon, mouse, pointer) paradigm, which is still heavily in use even in modern multitouch-based operating systems, we were able to develop an innovative new interface concept. Due to the use of the "cards" metaphor, and by focusing on tasks instead of applications, we were able to create a GUI which is both easier to understand and more enjoyable for elderly people than traditional computing environments.

2.3 Storyline

The Elisa UI is divided into three main sections: interests, friends and activities. For the realization of the three sections we followed a consistent card layout and concentrated on two different card layout variations. In the first out of three prototypes, both layouts were verified against the acceptance criteria among the tested users. In the end, a combination of the best layout concepts was chosen for implementation for the second prototype and improved for the third prototype.

For the interests and the activities sections, the content-centric layout was selected. The content-centric UI puts clear emphasis on displaying article content according to the users' personal interests. The user is invited to browse through daily updated articles and events of their preferred topics, according to the user's filter criteria. Contextually to the currently displayed articles and activities, the users are presented with the possibility to share the articles' contents with their family or friends or invite them to their personal events.

For the friends section, the person-centric layout was chosen emphasizing the social interaction between elderly people and their family or friends. The user is invited to browse through status messages, e-mails and shared photos. Users are supported in relationship building and staying in contact with family and friends. They can either send messages to their personal contacts, reply to e-mails or use Skype for voice or video conversations.

Providing the activity and content streams displayed in content-centric or person-centric layout remains a task executed in the background, invisible to the user. For this purpose the graphical layout is implemented as interactive android application communicating with the backend services provided by the Social Software Integration Layer and by additional web services.

Input methods for tablet computers
Modern tablet computers offer different input methods to generally control the device. Steve Jobs, founder of Apple Inc., is quoted naming the finger the best input method. His words were, however, clearly marketing talk, aimed at supporting Apple's business strategy with regard to products such as the iPhone and the iPad. In fact, our research shows that there is no "best input method" as every single one has its pros and cons. The most commonly used input methods for tablet computers nowadays are either the finger or the pen. While the finger is adequate for basic interactions like pushing a button it becomes less practical and sometimes even frustrating when it comes to more complex interactions such as handwriting. Furthermore, the finger needs a fairly large screen size in order to be accurate. This is especially important to consider when designing for elderly people. The pen on the other hand is a lot more precise and can even be used to digitize hand-writing and to perform other precision-needing tasks on tablet computers. A drawback is that the pen is one more device to carry around and limits the natural interaction and multi-touch functionality provided by touch based computers. As trembling hands are a common issue for elderly people, the pen is an optional but not an ideal input choice.

Typing on computers commonly happens with either an on-screen (virtual) or a physical keyboard. The physical keyboard is generally preferred by the user since it gives tactile feedback, a feature which is usually not included in an onscreen keyboard. A physical keyboard can be an external device attached to the tablet with a cable, connected wirelessly via Bluetooth or clicked into a docking station. Consequently, we considered both solutions for the Elisa device: a virtual on-screen keyboard as well as an optional attachable physical keyboard.

We have to point out that an on-screen keyboard has a bigger impact on the "screen real estate" of a graphical user interface than a hardware keyboard. The onscreen keyboard is either hiding graphical content by appearing on top of interactive elements or it triggers a change in the layout by stretching or resizing elements and content.

According to our assessments, input solutions such as voice recognition or hand-writing recognition have not yet reached the technical level required for our target group. They are often unresponsive, cumbersome to use and have high error rates. Hence, these features would most certainly produce a negative user experience.

In our opinion, the keyboard is the best choice for input as people are either familiar with computer keyboards or typewriters. However, results of the third prototype show, that the default virtual on-screen keyboards have to be adapted for elderly people. For example, automatic suggestions should be turned off, alternate settings should be hidden and all important characters should be displayed without the need of using the shift key.

Natural interaction support

Natural user interfaces (NUI) as multi-touch displays of tablet computers offer a new dimension of user interaction. Natural user interfaces are not a new technology, but rather a new human-computer interaction (HCI) technique that enables users to behave like in a natural environment, interacting with physical graspable/ tangible objects, haptics, gestures, hand writing and spoken natural language (Rauterberg et al. 1996). In 2008, August de los Reyes described NUI as the next evolutionary step from the desktop metaphor of today's GUI to direct manipulation of on-screen content and more intuitive interaction with computing systems (De los Reyes 2008).

Several ways of interactions with natural user interfaces exist, providing different levels of richness of interaction determined by the underlying technology. In the following sections, we distinguish between direct multi-touch interactions, indirect tangible interactions with physical objects and combined interactions with mobile and ubiquitous devices.

Touch interactions are mainly performed on graphical display surfaces or touchpads that track the position and movement of the hands or fingers of a user. Depending on the amount of concurrently recognizable fingers we also refer to single- or multi-touch surfaces. Modern touch interfaces enable users to perform gestures. In the domain of touch interaction, gestures are finger movements that are interpreted by the software application as commands, like panning or rotating virtual objects. Quick and simple gestures for navigation and editing are also called flicks.

Navigation and interaction patterns

The user experience very much depends on how intuitively a graphical user interface can be controlled or navigated. The user should be able to immediately distinguish between mere content and navigation elements that start an action. While there are different aspects that need to be considered, the placement of navigational objects is very important. On the other hand, these placements very much depend on the general form factor of the hardware and on how the user will interact with the device.

A tablet computer can either be held in the hand or placed on a table (using a stand) which means that the interaction may vary. Finger control is most commonly executed with the forefinger giving the user enough accuracy to point and hit the desired position on the screen. When holding the device with both hands, though, it is easier to use the thumbs.

The Elisa UI has been developed with the placement of the fingers in mind. The goal is to reduce the amount of hand-arm movement necessary to reach the desired elements on the screen, making the use of Elisa a less fatiguing experience. Even if the device is standing on a table, the suitable placement of interaction patterns and elements is important, although the areas are in that case arranged in a slightly different fashion.

We can assume that the user will tend to rest the arm on the table surface to prevent fatigue. Elderly people might become tired by holding up the arm for too long. To reach the upper part of the screen he or she has to raise the arm, so placing many elements there will produce a more tiring experience. Assuming that our user is right handed, he/she will have easier access to the areas closer to the resting position of the hand, which will assumedly be somewhere on the right side or central part of the tablet. We also need to keep in mind that resting the hand on the right side of the tablet will prevent obscuring the screen with the hand (or the arm) while interacting with the GUI. The user can interact with both hands though, so placing elements on the left side is also possible. Still the most important ones should be on the right side.

While creating the horizontal navigation, we had the accessible areas of both ergonomics in mind. Consequently, the navigational arrow buttons are located on the left and right sides of the screen. The most important navigational control is the next-page button as we assumed that the user wants to move to the next page more often than they want to go back to a previous page. Consequently for a right-handed person, this button is placed on the right, while the back button is placed on the left. On the vertical axis, both buttons are centered vertically, thus offering an ideal interaction, independently of how the user holds the device. While we mainly described the placement of elements for right-handed persons, we also had the needs of left-handed persons in mind. Those could be met by rearranging controls and elements such as the navigation or closing buttons.

Screen orientation

Modern tablet computers have the ability to seamlessly switch between landscape and portrait mode to ensure maximum flexibility according to the given content or application. While this technology can enhance the user experience, we believe that it would rather be conceived as disturbing or even confusing by our target group. To ensure consistency also in terms of graphical layout, we decided against this technology.

As a result, the landscape orientation was chosen since it can be considered a more "natural" orientation due to the screen ratio of 16:9 and the fact that it is similar to the format of an open book. From our experience, it is more comfortable holding a tablet computer in landscape mode than in portrait mode. This has been confirmed by our user tests in Spain and Germany.

As described in the section on content-centric layout, the decision for the landscape orientation resulted in a navigation following the horizontal plane. Therefore, the content can also be explored by using swipe gestures to move content to the right or left, that is, out of the screen.

Card layout

In our investigations, we analyzed user interface metaphors and paradigms currently used by manufacturers for desktop computers and tablets. The WIMP paradigm still is the standard for desktop computer interfaces (and of course also for their mobile counterparts, the notebook computers). Yet it was interesting to note that also tablet computers, which represent a major departure from how computers have worked until now, still use most of the conventions established by Xerox Parc in the seventies for their Alto computer. As previously noted, the whole desktop-icon paradigm, which we still find on iOS (iPhone Operating System) and android tablets, is functional for the business model that the systems relies on. It is vital for these systems to offer third party software developers the possibility to introduce additional software (so called apps) into the OS. This works fine for most people but makes the whole interface harder to use for the less experienced, since what a person wants to do when sitting in front of a computer is to perform a task and not to use an application.

For Elisa we wanted to concentrate just on the tasks the user wants to perform and remove all the unnecessary abstractions and metaphors we commonly find on modern operating systems, thus making the interface easier and more intuitive for elderly users. Accordingly displayed content and interactive elements are consistently presented inside rectangular frames, which we call "cards". These cards are like paper cards placed on an imaginary surface.

The card layout serves as simple and comprehensible metaphor for an information unit. For instance, a card can represent an article, a friend's message or an event summary. A simulated three dimensional representation of these cards (achieved by the use of drop shadows) helps differentiate between these interactive elements and the background, and further enhances the metaphor.

Cards can have different sizes, depending on the grid and the type of view the user chooses. Swiping a card to the left equals navigating to the next screen.

The physical movement of the cards communicates where the user is going in the interface. Moving a card to the right (or swiping the cards out of the left side of the screen) corresponds to advancing, while the contrary means going back to a previous step or page.

No icons are used to represent applications (there are no applications in the classical sense) or actions. Icons are only used to make text labels easier to understand and remember.

Animation

According to the results of deliverable 3.1 "End User Requirements" we avoided quick animations since the user most often cannot retrace the context changes and might feel lost or overwhelmed. On the other hand, when animations are kept simple and slow, they can be very helpful to help the user to better follow the navigation of the interface, like switching from one page to another or resizing content displayed on the screen.

Once the user is actively triggering an animation, for example by using a swipe gesture for switching between pages, he is capable of understanding and retracing it. The speed of the animations should be neither too fast nor too slow and ideally adapt to the preferred speed of the user. The main purpose of animations in Elisa is to guide the elderly users along the performed steps and prevent confusion and disorientation.

In conclusion we are using animations to support the elderly in understanding the horizontal navigation concept. The placement of the two arrow buttons on each sides of the screen also corresponds to this animation concept, since their position is connected with the physical movement of the central screen contents.

Adaptive user interface

The Elisa UI is designed to become an adaptive user interface. The idea is to take the user's technical experience into consideration and only offer simple functionalities for beginners. Based on the users' behavior the Elisa UI will gradually unlock functionalities as the user becomes familiar with the existing functionality. Once a new feature is available the user gets a hint and can watch a tutorial video explaining how to use the new functionality. Afterwards, the user can decide for or against the use of that functionality.

We would like to point out that there are various aspects that could eventually lead to an adaptive user interface. At this stage, we only conceptualized the adaptive user interface and decided to concentrate on the full implementation of the UI first. We suggest elaborating the adaptive UI in the end product.

Adaptive user interface

The design has been unified using a common layout grid for all areas. This grid is based on the overview page of each section and helps to improve the visual consistency throughout the interface. The upper part of the screen is reserved for general information (e.g. date, battery status and time) as well as the action tab that gives the user access to basic help functionalities (Fig. 9). The height of the arrow

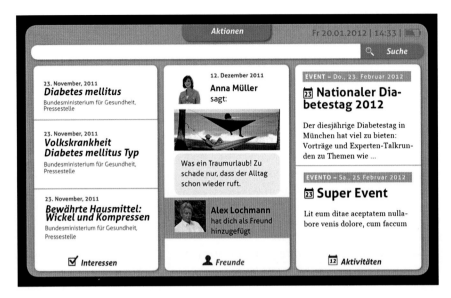

Fig. 9 Start page—main content screen with overview about latest articles, messages and upcoming events

buttons on both sides of the screen matches the size of the central content field and the arrows are big enough to be pressed by the elderly from different angles regardless of the way the device is held.

In each section, the content is displayed in chronological order. The user can use the arrow buttons to navigate back and forth between different pages and the back button to return to previous sections. The three tab buttons at the bottom of the screen represent the entry point for the management layer. We decided to place the tab buttons at the bottom to ensure that they will not be pressed by accident or interfere with the horizontal navigation (see the section on screen orientation).

The interests section is like an interactive magazine and is based on a three column grid offering the user the possibility to browse and choose content according to their personal interests. By selecting any of the displayed content, the user is able to read the content in full-screen mode. The content type is divided into several categories, like articles, events/activities, photo streams or status messages from friends and family members.

In the article's detail view, depending on the length of the article, the content will be split among as many pages (cards) as needed. Using the arrow buttons (or a simple swipe gesture) the user can navigate between cards. We decided to spread longer content over several pages instead of keeping it on one page so the user does not need to scroll, an activity that has proven to be more complicated for the elderly to manage. An additional interaction element is the timeline bar just below the article content. The timeline bar provides a clue on how many pages are available and it is designed as interactive navigation control.

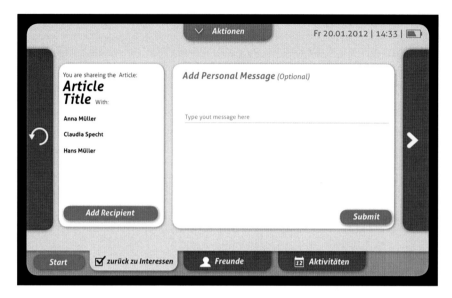

Fig. 10 Interests section—article sharing functionality is shown in action bar according to the current context

Content can also be shared with friends or family contacts via e-mail in order to trigger an active discussion. In addition to sharing an article's contents the user can add a personal message to the article (Fig. 10).

Instead of a calendar replacement we developed a completely new social calendar based on the card layout for the activities section. The social calendar in Elisa allows the user to save events and to discover new events based on suggestions of the system as well as on the user-selected categories. Thus we obtained a comprehensible overview of events and simplified the browsing for elderly users.

Person-centric layout

The person-centric layout of the friends section emphasizes the social interaction with acquaintances, friends, relatives or contacts with same interests, e.g. from a sports club or cooking course. The intention is to stay aware of what (remotely living) family members and friends are doing. Part of the social interaction is to actively share information with other people or comment on provided content.

For this purpose information from different Social Networking Services is accessed and aggregated by the Social Software Integration Layer (SSIL) and presented in the Elisa UI frontend. Due to the consistent design and data aggregation techniques the data sources and the data retrieval processes of the SSIL remain hidden from the user.

The friends section's overview page provides a different functionality in comparison to the activities section. It serves as a social activity stream of the Elisa user's contacts, presented in the compact and consistent card layout (see the section on card layout). The Elisa UI presents Facebook/Google+ posts, e-mails, photos shared and articles all in the same look-and-feel. The user can read and reply to messages and does not have to think about the communication channel. The SSIL handles incoming messages, creates new users and manages the communication.

Using the input field on top of the page the user will be able to write a message that will be visible to all contacts. The first card offers the possibility to access the address book and browse through the contacts. The main screen shows the most recent activities from people on the contact list in inverse chronological order. The browsing of the messages is performed on a horizontal axis. By clicking on a person the user accesses the profile view which presents the personal details and all activities of this particular person. The profile view follows the card layout, a first card showing a photo of the person and offering up to three buttons to send e-mails or perform voice or video calls in case the person is available online (shown by a green checkmark). The second card shows all available information on a contact, such as the contact's address, telephone number and hobbies. An additional interactive interaction element is the timeline bar just below the content stream.

References

De los Reyes, A.: Predicting the past, A Design Vision for Microsoft Surface. Microsoft (2008)

Rauterberg, M., Stebler, R., Mauch, T.: Augmented reality in contest with a command, desktop and touch screen interface. In: Proceedings of 5th International Conference INTERFACE to Real & Virtual World (1996)

System Development Frontend: How We Developed and Integrated the Elisa Software

Wilhelm Prasser and Marc Delling

1 Executive Summary

At the very beginning of the project one idea was to develop a simple application (AppStore approach) for downloading from one of the Standard AppStores powered by Apple or Google. But during our analysis of the requirements supported by the focus groups, internal testing and research, we quickly recognized that the desired features and functionalities could not be implemented with a simple App-based graphical user interface (GUI) approach. The flexibility and capabilities standard software development kits provided were by far not powerful enough to fulfil our needs.

So we took the hard way and developed a completely new GUI adapted to the specific needs of our target audience replacing the Standard Android GUI (Start Screen).

2 Main Results

Android allows replacing the standard GUI with an alternative GUI during the boot procedure via the boot setup (Launcher). Thus, our idea was to distribute the development over different stages of the prototypes, each should be tested with a certain holistic feedback loop with the dedicated user groups. The results should engender improvements and requirements for the next stage of the prototype. With this approach we checked the acceptance of and also reduced the complexity for the elderly by asking only for feedback on certain experiences without overwhelming them with too many technology features.

W. Prasser (✉)
Data United GmbH, Munich, Germany
e-mail: wilhelm.prasser@data-united.de

M. Delling
Silpion IT-Solutions GmbH, Hamburg, Germany

E. F. Moritz (ed.), *Assistive Technologies for the Interaction of the Elderly*,
Advanced Technologies and Societal Change, DOI: 10.1007/978-3-319-00678-9_7,
© Springer International Publishing Switzerland 2014

3 Storyline

Apart from all the "standard" challenges during a software development process, we faced additional requirements in this specific project which are simply caused by the specific user group (and their needs), the dedicated GUI design (design meets technology) and the limited support provided by the Standard Android SDK (especially for non-standard features).

One of the hurdles especially was in the area of text handling, views building and animation features. For example, Android does not provide any feature for handling text blocks, which means that we needed to develop our own function-alities to break text into several columns. State of the art within Android is to frame text to a certain width an then provide a scroll-function with a variable height, but in our GUI we had a fixed frame with a defined height and width. Moreover, Android is not even able to provide a function telling you the amount of text which has already been displayed. We needed to build all these missing functionalities and moreover discovered that text rendering can sometimes have a lot of bugs and is thus not really reliable (Fig. 1).

We know that we challenged the SDK quite a lot with some unusual require-ments like paging (here, text rendering plays a certain role as well) and with splitting the screen into different frames (fragments), but we needed these features for the individual animations within the screen. Based on this unusual screen layout, the fragment classes were blown up to so-called monster-classes, which are all structured somehow but include quite a large amount of functionalities.

3.1 Development Phases

The development team consisted of two core members, two associate members and a supervisor. The team interacted and coordinated itself by using a KanBan-style task board and daily stand-up meetings. To keep all team members in sync, every prototype iteration was introduced with a vision statement.

As mentioned before, we distributed the development process over the three prototype stages, each defined with a dedicated goal and with certain functionalities.

Elisa prototype I vision statement: For the development team, Elisa prototype I is a technology demonstrator that shows the feasibility of the Elisa graphical user interface and the view transition which can be animated smoothly. It should help the team with the decision process concerning the further Elisa prototype development.

Apart from the vision statement, a task board and stand-up-meetings were performed on a regular basis. There were, however, no additional project man-agement tools used in the development phase for prototype I.

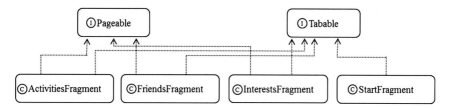

Fig. 1 Core elements

For the appropriate view transitions, Android Animators are used. They are classes that can be fitted to any Android view class and can be used to do timed transformations on their properties (translate, rotate, scale). Furthermore the resulting Animators could then be grouped in standard collections and handed to an AnimatorSet, which then controls the whole animator ensemble; for instance all animations can be played at the same time or one at a time.

Elisa prototype II vision statement: For the target audience—elderly people— the Elisa prototype II was designed as a mock-up information assistant showing the Elisa user interface and animated view transitions in strict compliance to a given test protocol. In addition to the Elisa prototype I, the users could really see a certain look-and-feel of what could be expected of the Elisa GUI.

Prototype II had a strict testing scenario. All tasks were entered as tickets in Redmine (Project Management Tool in Phase 2) and processed accordingly. Most of the additional external team collaboration was also handled via Redmine. Additionally, each development team member received a set of cards containing the test-scenarios developed by the UniBwM team, and the developers were encouraged to test the scenarios on a regular basis to make sure everything ran smoothly and as expected.

Elisa prototype III vision statement: For the elderly, the Elisa prototype III was an interactive information assistant. In addition to the Elisa prototype II, users could share activities, use interacting gestures and focus on specific interests of their own (profiling).

Prototype III included an extensive workload of screen-design, screen-inter-actions and refactoring of all animations. Extensive work had to be done in the handling of text, text views and pages, because Android requires customization for the animated card layout for user-interface concepts that deviate from those pro-vided by the Android system as standards. To cope with this kind of workload, the focus shifted from the task board to a "wallpaper" of printouts of all screens. Tasks associated with screens were directly attached to it with blue sticky notes. Sticky notes with other colors were used to give additional information or to highlight problems and impediments.

With the integration of the real backend with a classic relational database model, the need for an object-relational mapper on Android emerged—a layer that fills the gap between the database and the presented information. Because this mapping is an error-prone process, it is advised to use automated tools or a well-tested framework to perform the work. There are various such frameworks available for Android and two were taken into further consideration:

ORMLite is an object-relational mapper for Android and SQLite that had been used before in various projects and had proven to be quite usable. ORMLite uses annotations like other Java-persistence frameworks in enterprise systems (JPA, Hibernate) to map database-models to model classes.

GreenDAO uses code generation techniques to build model-classes and integrate functions to fill them with database information. It can be expected that GreenDAO might be faster than ORMLite because its data model is generated instead of mapped, but the lack of available information on this specific topic made it an uncertain decision.

We decided in favour of ORMLite because it is a more mature and stable product compared to GreenDAO and the mapping using annotations is more convenient and better known in the Java developer community.

At the end of the day and with great support by UniBwM, we managed to provide and launch the final prototype and performed the testing in Spain and in Germany with the user groups. Their feedback was quite positive and we now know exactly what they expect from the final product. But before we go there, we want to describe the software architecture in more detail.

3.2 Software Architecture: Core Elements

In the following section, we describe the elements which were used for the software architecture and their functionalities

The four main views (start, interests, friends and activities) were implemented as fragments, as advised by the best practices for Android 4.0. To introduce the needed behavior for Android we developed the interfaces "pageable" for fragments which include content covering several pages. We also created "tabable" for all fragments that needed to be alternated by some sort of tab controller.

The key design pattern was of course the ubiquitous model view controller (MVC) pattern. It was vital during the development process to get it right the first time, because later on, the UniBwM team implemented the integration of the backend for the prototype III.

For some features, third party libraries where used. Here the licensing had to be considered and therefore we only used libraries which also were useable for commercial use (Apache, MIT, BSD) and didn't require a full disclosure of source code.

For the so-called lazy-loading of images, the Shutterbug library was used and, as already mentioned before, ORMLite as object-relational database mapper.

We would like to highlight some additional comments:

No Android standard user interface elements were used, so all visual elements were customized.

If a newly designed user interface element was needed, the visual component of the element was created using 9-Patch PNGs. These are special PNGs where the four corners, four edges and the middle area (together nine elements, thus the naming) are distinguishable regions of the image and therefore can be handled independently when resizing. The corners will be immutable while the edges scale in one axis and the middle in both.

3.3 Summary

We think we achieved a great result in the development process of the GUI. Apart from all the challenges we faced during the different stages, we see it as a great benefit to develop something like the Elisa user interface more or less from scratch. Getting so much input and feedback during the different phases of the process (user groups, backend experts and designers) it is not easy to say "this will never work" because the expectations were quite high and so we had to find ways to "tell" the device, the SDK and also the program code what exactly it was we wanted to implement.

One of the biggest advantages during the project were the participating partners because they were always willing to discuss things again and again until we found a way in which it could work and also a result which was accepted by the different stakeholders.

Social Software Integration: How We Made Social Software Services Accessible

Martin Burkhard, Andrea Nutsi and Michael Koch

1 Executive Summary

For supplying elderly people with an activity and content feed that offers information on what is happening in their community and local environment, an information and communication infrastructure has to be provided that integrates Social Networking Services (SNS) including Social Networks, photo sharing sites, address book services, personal blogs, web feeds and mailing lists. In this section, we present our approach to integrating existing SNS and facilitating social interaction for the elderly.

2 Main Results

In the AAL project SI-Screen/Elisa, our core goal was to support social interaction by making services from the Social Web available to the elderly. As part of the Social Web, Social Network sites (e.g. Facebook^{TM}, Google+^{TM} etc.) and photo sharing communities (e.g. Flickr^{TM}, Picasa^{TM}, etc.) are web-based platforms for building online communities by establishing social ties between individuals (Boyd and Ellison 2007). In the following, we use the broader term Social Networking Services (SNS) to also consider Web 2.0 websites like blogs or wikis that enable individuals to publish and share content as well as interact with each other.

Figure 1 shows the current state of how tablet devices like the Apple iPad^{TM} or Android^{TM} tablet computers can be used to participate in the Social Web. Third party companies develop so-called rich client applications (apps) that handle the access to SNS in the Web. The advantage of this approach is that missing software components and functionalities can be added over time. The drawback of this

M. Burkhard (✉) · A. Nutsi · M. Koch
Universität der Bundeswehr München, Neubiberg, Germany
e-mail: martin.burkhard@unibw.de

E. F. Moritz (ed.), *Assistive Technologies for the Interaction of the Elderly*,
Advanced Technologies and Societal Change, DOI: 10.1007/978-3-319-00678-9_8,
© Springer International Publishing Switzerland 2014

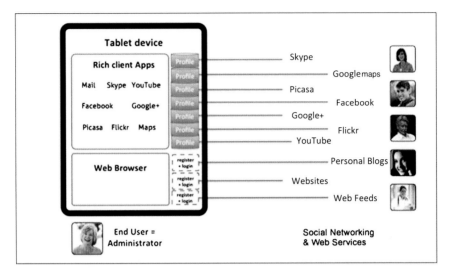

Fig. 1 Current state of tablet computer—for every SNS, a separate rich client app exists. Photos licensed by Fotolia

solution is that every app has its own non-consistent graphical layout and for access to most services the end user has to register and login separately to access each service. Apart from that, a web browser can be used to access services—again with inconsistent user interfaces and separate user accounts.

Eventually, an elderly user would have to take over the administrative tasks like registering user accounts as well as installing and updating applications on their own. In our focus group sessions we found out that elderly people hesitate to create an account to participate in online communities of SNS (Burkhard and Koch 2012). These findings are also supported by (Brucks and Reckin 2012), pointing out that apps on existing tablet devices are too difficult to be understood and used by elderly users. Moreover, currently users of one online community are not able to easily participate in the community of another web platform (Burkhard and Koch 2012).

The main result of this part of the project is giving elderly people universal access to SNS without the need to deal with the underlying technical details. For this purpose, we introduced the Social Software Integration Layer (SSIL, Fig. 2) that uses CommunityMashup (Lachenmaier et al. 2012) to provide every elderly Elisa user with a combined information stream of consolidated contact profiles and aggregated activity and content streams originating from different SNS platforms (see Sect. 4). The advantage of a combined information stream for the elderly users is that instead of maintaining several dispersed online communities, the single information stream will give them the impression of taking part in only one homogeneous community (Burkhard and Koch 2012). And due to a consistent layout of the Elisa frontend, the various information sources will remain hidden to the (elderly) users (Nutsi et al. 2013). In addition to the already existing

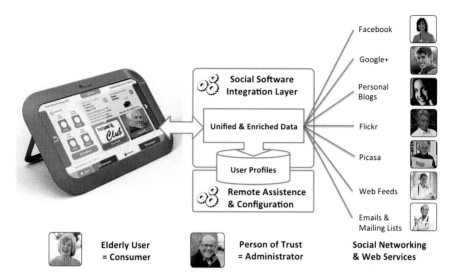

Fig. 2 Elisa—the Social Software Integration Layer provides elderly Elisa users with universal access to SNS. Photos licensed by Fotolia

CommunityMashup adaptors for Facebook and email servers, we also added support for the integration of different sources for contacts, images, events and blogs.

Within the scope of the SI-Screen/Elisa project, we created two web applications to relieve the Elisa users from administrative tasks such as account registration or social network management required by every SNS: The Profile Admin User Interface (Profile Admin UI, see Fig. 5) that enables the delegation of administrative tasks to a person of trust; and the Channel User Interface (Channel UI) that provides an interface for friends and family contacts of the elderly Elisa users to proactively give access to their activity and content streams.

3 Storyline

Social Networking Services (SNS) like Facebook, Google+ and Flickr serve as platforms for fostering social networks with relatives and friends or for establishing social relationships with new people online. In the last years, people worldwide started sharing their real-life activities and feelings via status messages and photos, finding like-minded people and learning about events in the vicinity. Elderly people, however, are still often excluded from these interactions as they face several technical barriers.

The first obstacle of becoming a member of an online community is the mandatory registration process that usually requires an existing email account and a memorable password. This registration is often followed by the set-up of a personal profile by providing personal information like date of birth, gender, location, as well as personal information on family and friends.

Another obstacle is the missing interconnectivity of SNS platforms. While members of online communities form connected groups within one SNS platform, they are unable to connect and communicate with online communities on other SNS platforms. Thus, the same registration process and the continuous management of one's identity and personal network have to be performed for every SNS all over again. This administrative overhead is not just a burden for elderly people with low technical affinity, but also outweighs the unacquainted benefits.

Another aspect is the growing concern regarding privacy in SNS. Elderly people are well aware of ongoing debates in media about privacy and security issues in social networks (see the paragraph on "Data privacy and information security"). This often discourages them from registering at SNS. Consequently, avoiding a direct registration in SNS and gaining and keeping the elderlies' trust by protecting their personal data is key to the success of the Elisa product.

In summary, elderly people could profit from the advantages of SNS by overcoming the barriers outlined. As a result of the SI-Screen/Elisa project, our contribution regarding this issue was to make SNS more accessible for elderly people by abstracting from the underlying technology and delegating administrative tasks to a person of trust. As a consequence, the Elisa users do not even have to register and maintain a profile to take part in existing online communities. How this is achieved is explained in more detail in the following paragraphs.

Technological challenges

Throughout the project, we faced the technological challenge of integrating activity and content streams from heterogeneous SNS, which usually have proprietary data structures, vary in authentication and authorization methods, and offer Web application programming interfaces (Web APIs, see Sect. 4) that change over time. So instead of integrating SNS directly into the Elisa tablet client software, we opted for a distributed client server approach which has the advantage that the integration of new SNS or changes in existing SNS APIs only result in server-side adaptions, while the Elisa tablet client remains unaffected. In other words, elderly Elisa users benefit from new content and SNS support without having to update their tablet devices.

Social Software Integration Layer

Our solution for the server-side part of Elisa was the Social Software Integration Layer (SSIL). For building the SSIL, we had to find a scalable middleware solution that is capable of aggregating user profiles and combining activity and content streams from several sources, thus producing personalized results (mashups). Ideally, the SSIL should synchronize data with SNS and other non-social third-party web services using pluggable components allowing on-the-fly adaptions without maintenance shut-downs. Moreover, the SSIL solution has to support filtering operations and do secure synchronization with mobile devices.

The analysis of existing solutions for the implementation of the SSIL and the possibilities for integrating semi-structured information residing on web sites can be found in the Scientific Excursion (Sect. 4). The Social Software Integration Layer (SSIL) is software that runs on a server computer on the Internet. The server

Table 1 External Social Networking Services (SNS) integrated by the Social Software Integration Layer (SSIL)

Service	Integration contents	Service type
Google Contacts	Profile data (name, e-mail, address, photo, Skype-account)	Contacts service
Facebook	Profile data (name, e-mail, photo), status messages (text, photo)	Social community service
Google+	Profile data (name, e-mail, photo), status messages (text, photo)	Social community service
Google Picasa	Images	Image service
Yahoo! Flickr	Images	Image service
Elisa Magazine	Text, images, categories, tags	Syndicate feed
Event web sites (RSS)	Text, images, start, end, location	Syndicate feed
Personal blogs	Text, images	Blog service/syndicate feed
Mailing lists	Text, images	Email service

enables end user software on mobile devices to access several SNS and other data sources in a unified way. For this purpose, the SSIL unifies the profile data, activity streams (status updates) and content streams (comments, recommendations, photos) of existing SNS (Facebook, Google+), social content sharing platforms (Flickr, Picasa), contact management (Google Contacts^{TM}) as well as web feeds (events, articles), mailing lists and personal blogs. The complete list of services integrated in the Elisa prototype with some more details is shown in Table 1.

Figure 3 shows that the SSIL serves several users at once but still maintains strictly separate instances for every user. The SSIL does not have a particular user interface. Instead, the SSIL provides end user applications on mobile devices with a secure, unified bi-directional access to unified and enriched data via an application programming interface. To this end, the SSIL uses an individual configuration for each Elisa user containing user account information and authorization information for access to the activity and content streams of integrated SNS. The set-up of new user account profiles can be managed by a system administrator using the MashupConfigurator, as can be seen in Fig. 4. As part of the SSIL, the Profile Admin UI (Fig. 5) offers a remote support web interface which enables a person of trust (e.g. a family member or friend) to assist in case of problems or take over the administrative tasks from the elderly user. These administrative tasks include the management of the user's profile, personal contacts and device settings:

- Start: overview of opened and closed help requests.
- Elisa User Management: Adapt contact details of the Elisa user like address, telephone and hobbies.
- Contact Management: Add or edit contacts and assign them to contact groups.
- Settings: Adjust tablet-specific settings remotely.
- Filter Categories: Modify user's interests by remotely filtering content of the "interests" and "activities" sections.
- Password Management: Reset the password of an Elisa user.

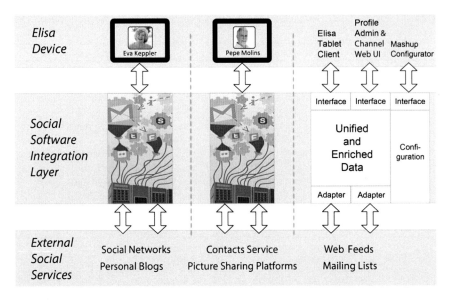

Fig. 3 Elisa Architecture—Elisa tablets, the Social Software Integration Layer and external SNS integration. Image based on Lachenmaier et al. (2012). Photos licensed by Fotolia

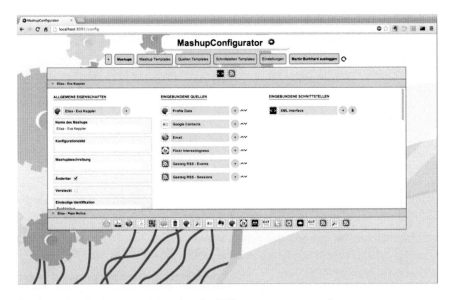

Fig. 4 MashupConfigurator—Managing the SNS source components for every user

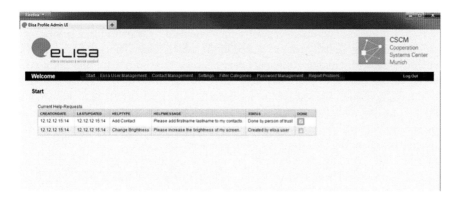

Fig. 5 Elisa Profile Admin UI—Menu and overview listing help requests

Moreover, the person of trust can use the Profile Admin UI to invite family members and friends to authorize Elisa users to access their personal Facebook, Google+, Flickr and/or Picasa activity and content streams. As part of this invitation, the email contact receives a personalized link to the Elisa Channel UI web interface and a one-time password. Subsequently, the invitee uses his or her email address and the one-time password to log into the Channel UI forcing them to select a personal password after their first authentication.

After the successful login, the main screen of the Elisa Channel UI provides an overview of supported SNS channels from which the invitees can select the channels they would like to share with a single Elisa user. Selecting a SNS channel starts an authorization process, during which the invitee authenticates and approves the SNS access. This authorization is valid for a given amount of time depending on the SNS. At any time, the invitee can log in again and either withdraw previous authorization or grant access to additional channels.

In the end, the Elisa user has access to all authorized activity and content streams without being a member of the underlying SNS. Moreover, the SSIL ensures bi-directional communication between the mobile tablet client and the external service (see Figs. 3, 8 and 9).

Backend filtering

Combining activity and content feeds from (highly) active online communities and information services results in an increasing amount of information delivered to the Elisa user. In order to prevent the risk of information overload (Hiltz and Turoff 1985) and considering the limited bandwidth of mobile clients, the SSIL provides filtering mechanisms controlling what content is processed from external SNS and what information is forwarded to the user.

On the one hand, the MashupConfigurator allows system administrators to configure the frequency, kind and amount of information collected from various external SNS sources. On the other hand, the Elisa client can pass combinable filter criteria to the synchronization point (REST interface, see Lachenmaier et al. 2011, 2012) to narrow down the search results.

For example, during the field test, the email adapter checked for new messages every five minutes. The messages were then checked by a spam filter before their contents were aggregated and forwarded to the tablet client. The address book was synchronized with Google Contacts every 15 min. Due to our limited amount of articles for the field test, every day up to three articles from the Elisa magazine and up to three activities were shown to the elderly user. Each article and activity was assigned to one out of five categories. These categories serve as selectable filter criteria for the elderly user in the Elisa frontend enabling adjustment of the information provided according to their personal interests.

For the Elisa product, an increase in amount of articles and information from SNS is to be expected. To accept this challenge our intention is to combine the individual selected filter criteria and browsing behavior to derive a filtering profile for information filtering (Belkin and Croft 1992). This filtering profile is collected in the Elisa client device and transferred to the SSIL to prioritize and filter content of integrated information streams of external SNS. For this purpose we looked into recommender systems (Resnick and Varian 1997) and ranking algorithms (Koroleva and Bolufé Röhler 2012) currently used by Social Network sites.

Data privacy and information security
Processing personal data requires compliance with data privacy laws and regulations of Germany and Spain in which the Elisa clients are located and the SSIL server is hosted. Accordingly, the European Data Protection Directives (95/46/EC,[1] 2002/58/EC3,[2] 2006/25/EC[3]), the German Federal Data Protection Act and the Telecommunications Act, as well as the Spanish Royal Decree 1720/2007 apply.

Against this background, the Organization for Economic Co-operation and Development (OECD) defined the "Basic Principles of National Application".[4] In the following we summarize the main aspects:

- Collection Limitation Principle: The amount of collected data should be limited.
- Data Quality Principle: Personal data should be relevant, necessary, accurate and complete.
- Purpose Specification Principle: The purpose of the collected data should be specified.
- Use Limitation Principle: Personal data should not be disclosed or made available.

[1] European Directive 95/46/EC on the protection of individuals with regard to the processing of personal data and on the free movement of such data.

[2] European Directive 2002/58/EC concerning the processing of personal data and the protection of privacy in the electronic communications sector (Directive on privacy and electronic communications).

[3] European Directive 2006/24/EC on the retention of data generated or processed in connection with the provision of publicly available electronic communications services or of public communications networks and amending.

[4] OECD—Basic Principles of National Application. Available: http://www.oecd.org/internet/ ieconomy/oecdguidelinesontheprotectionofprivacyandtransborderflowsofpersonaldata.htm.

- Security Safeguards Principle: Personal data should be protected by security measurements.
- Openness Principle: general policy of openness with respect to the existence and nature of personal data, the purpose of their use and the identity of the data controller.
- Individual Participation Principle: the right of individuals to get confirmation in time if the data controller has data related to them and to have data erased, rectified, completed or amended.
- Accountability Principle: The data controller should be accountable for complying with data privacy measures.

Following the collection limitation principle, the SSIL server only stores authentication information required to access the personal email account and external SNS of the Elisa user in the CommunityMashup configuration file. In addition, we store the email address, a hashed password and SNS authentication information for the person of trust and every invitee. Personal data collected from the email server and external SNS is processed but not stored on the server's hard disk.

In the SI-Screen/Elisa project, we use a combination of information security measurements in compliance with the Security Safeguards principle to protect personal data against unauthorized disclosure or access:

- For every Elisa user we run a strictly separated SSIL server instance and offer individual Profile Admin and Channel UI web sites (Fig. 3).
- Communication between the Elisa tablet client and the SSIL backend is protected by the HTTPS protocol for secure communication.
- OAuth 2.0 authentication and authorization infrastructure ensures that only Elisa users have access to their personal synchronization endpoint.
- At the operating system level, we rely on secure hosting services (e.g. encryption, firewall) of the hosting Internet service provider.

4 Scientific Excursion

In the next sections, we present the web application programming interfaces (Web APIs) and content aggregation technologies we analyzed for the design of the Social Software Integration Layer (SSIL) and the types of data sources we integrated.

Web APIs
A prerequisite for integrating external Social Networking Services (SNS) is that SNS providers allow third-party developers to use their web-based services by offering a machine-to-machine communication interface, also known as Web API. A Web API specifies how the server processes requests and responses as well as the structure of the data exchanged during communication.

Table 2 Selected Web APIs for common social services including their authentication models, protocols and data interchange formats

Web API	Authentication/authorization models	Communication protocols	Data interchange formats
Facebook Graph API	OAuth 2.0, OpenID	REST	JSON
Google Contacts API	AuthSub, ClientLogin, OpenID, OAuth, (OAuth2.0[a])	GData, Atom	GData, Atom, JSON
Google Plus API	AuthSub, ClientLogin, OpenID, OAuth, (OAuth2.0[a])	GData, Atom	GData, Atom, JSON
Google Picasa API	AuthSub, ClientLogin, OpenID, OAuth, (OAuth2.0[a])	GData, Atom	GData, Atom, JSON
Wordpress API	OAuth 2.0	REST, XML-RPC	XML, JSON
Yahoo! Flickr API	API key, OpenID, BBAuth, OAuth	REST, SOAP, XML-RPC	XML, JSON

[a] Experimental implementation

Today, an increasing number of SNS platforms provide a publicly available Web API. However, due to missing standards these Web APIs differ in extensiveness and quality. As a consequence, we had to analyze existing Web APIs against end-user requirements. Table 2 presents the examined Web APIs of supported SNS and gives an overview of the common authentication and authorization methods, the communication protocols and the formats used for data interchange. For implementation, we preferred the most common OAuth 2.0 authentication standard in combination with Representational State Transfer (REST) communication protocol and the data interchange format JavaScript Object Notation (JSON).

Content aggregation technologies

To realize the SSIL, we analyzed existing aggregation technologies, including available mashup services with regard to their matching of the requirements of Elisa. Table 3 lists the examined content aggregation technologies for mash-up solutions supporting the integration of external web services or feeds. The applied categorization is based on the classification model by Hoyer and Fischer (2008). Let's have a look at them.

Yahoo! Pipes[TM] service is a visual web tool that enables the combination of heterogeneous web services into a mash-up solution. Web resources, e.g. web feeds, are added as data source components which are linked by "pipes" for data aggregation and manipulation, see also Fig. 6. The data processing wiring by "pipes" is comparable to the UNIX shell pipeline concept. In principle Yahoo! Pipes could serve as solution for realizing the SSIL. However, this service leaves no control of where and how the private data would be processed by its servers. Most probably the location of the servers is outside of the European Union.

Yahoo! Dapper[TM] is a Software-as-a-Service (SaaS) tool for generating dynamic web feeds (e.g. RSS, Atom, JSON, XML, iCal). Dapper allows the extraction of dynamic content from any web site to be used as dynamic feed, see also Fig. 7.

Table 3 List of analyzed content aggregation technologies for Elisa backend service integration

Aggregator	Functionality/property	Target group	Features	Platform
ARIS MeshZone™	Presentation, adapter	Enterprise	Charts and diagrams based on Excel, CSV, XML data	Local web application
CommunityMashup	Transformation/aggregation, adapter	Consumer/ Enterprise	Middleware, person-centric data aggregation	Equinox (OSGi) solution, EMF editor
IBM Mashup Center™	Adapter, repository	Enterprise	Integrates with Infosphere and Lotus Notes	Local web application
JackBe Presto™	Transformation/aggregation, presentation	Enterprise	Service definition based on *EMML*, *jQuery*	Remote web application
Serena Business Mashups™	Presentation	Enterprise	Process-based IT Service Management	Local desktop application
Yahoo! Pipes™	Transformation/aggregation, repository	Consumer/ Enterprise	Unix pipe like aggregation of data provided by web feeds	Remote web application
Yahoo! Dapper	Adapter, repository	Consumer/ Enterprise	Web site data mapper and feed publisher	Remote web application

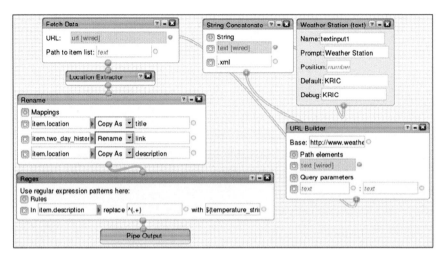

Fig. 6 Yahoo! PipesTM—enables the visual composition and aggregation of web resources. *Image source* Yahoo! PipesTM

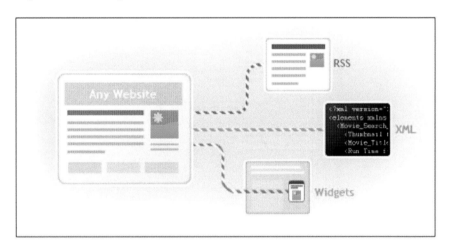

Fig. 7 Yahoo! DapperTM—produces dynamic web feeds based on web site content. *Image source* Yahoo! DapperTM

This includes web search results and dynamic table elements. In fact, Yahoo! Dapper does not fulfill the needs for creating the SSIL. Nevertheless, this service is very useful for extracting semi-structured data, for example from event web sites that do not offer a web feed or API.

CommunityMashup[5] is an open source social software middleware solution developed by Peter Lachenmaier et al. (2011, 2012). It provides a people-centric

---

[5] CommunityMashup—available: https://github.com/soziotech/CommunityMashup

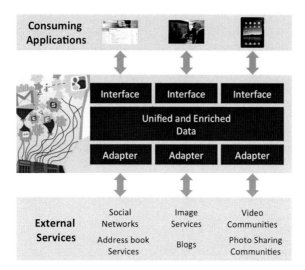

Fig. 8 CommunityMashup—aggregates data from Social Networking Services using a person-centric approach. *Image source* (Lachenmaier et al. 2012)

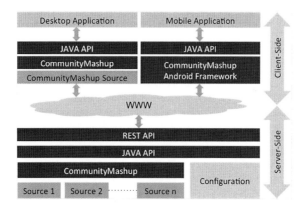

Fig. 9 CommunityMashup—Distributed environment with source components handling communication with Web APIs of external services. *Image source* (Lachenmaier et al. 2012)

approach for aggregating data from SNS and uses a service-oriented architecture (SOA) to integrate existing SNS and web feeds as pluggable service components (Figs. 8 and 9). In addition, the CommunityMashup framework supports common desktop, Web and mobile client platforms including Android™, iOS™, Windows Phone™ as well as HTML and JavaScript. CommunityMashup uses Equinox,[6] an

---

[6] Equinox—an implementation of the OSGi R4 core framework specification. Available: http://www.eclipse.org/equinox/

OSGi[7] runtime environment. As a consequence, new functionalities and data sources can be added as Java[TM]-based OSGi plug-ins on-the-fly[8] without the need to update the client code or shutting down the server for maintenance.

Our findings showed that ARIS MeshZone[TM], IBM Mashup center[TM], JackBe Presto[TM] and Serena Business Mashups[TM] do not meet our requirements as they lack the integration of the Web APIs of existing SNS. They mainly support XML and/or web feeds and focus on enterprise-specific business needs, like generating charts, diagrams, or workflows.

In the end, we decided to use CommunityMashup as the core of the Social Software Integration Layer in combination with Yahoo! Dapper[TM] in order to extract semi-structured content from web sites without public Web API.

References

Belkin, N.J., Croft, W.B.: Information filtering and information retrieval: two sides of the same coin? Commun. ACM **35**, 29–38 (1992). doi:10.1145/138859.138861

Boyd, D.M., Ellison, N.B.: Social network sites: definition, history, and scholarship. J. Comput.-Mediat. Commun. **13**, 210–230 (2007). doi:10.1111/j.1083-6101.2007.00393.x

Brucks, M., Reckin, R.: Ist das iPad fit für Ältere? In: Reiterer, H., Deussen, O. (eds.) Proceedings of the Mensch und Computer 2012. Oldenbourg Verlag, (2012) pp. 45–51

Burkhard, M., Koch, M.: Social Interaction Screen. Making Social Networking Services Accessible for Elderly People. i-com 11, pp. 3–7 (2012). doi: 10.1524/icom.2012.0030

Hiltz, S., Turoff, M.: Structuring computer-mediated communication systems to avoid information overload. Commun. ACM **28**, 680–689 (1985)

Hoyer, V., Fischer, M.: Market overview of enterprise Mashup tools. In: Proceedings of the 6th International Conference on Service-Oriented Computing. Springer, Berlin, (2008) pp. 708–721

Koroleva, K., Bolufé Röhler, A.J.: Reducing information overload: design and evaluation of filtering & ranking algorithms for social network sites. Proceedings of the 20th European Conference on Information Systems (ECIS 2012), (2012) pp. 1–6

Lachenmaier, P., Ott, F.: Building a person-centric mashup system. communityMashup: A service oriented approach. In: Eichhorn D, Koschmider A, Zhang H (eds.) Proceedings of the 3rd Central-European Workshop on Services and their Composition (ZEUS 2011). CEUR-WS.org, Karlsruhe, Germany, pp. 122–129 (2011)

Lachenmaier, P., Ott, F., Koch, M.: Model-driven development of a person-centric mashup for social software. Soc. Netw. Anal. Min, online fir:1–15 (2012). doi: 10.1007/s13278-012-0064-x

Nutsi, A., Burkhard, M., Koch, M.: Providing access to social networking services for elderly people. Proceedings of Human Computer Interaction International (HCII) (2013)

Resnick, P., Varian, HR.: Recommender systems. Commun. ACM **40**:56–58 (1997). doi: 10.1145/245108.245121

---

[7] OSGi[TM]—a dynamic module system for Java[TM]. Available: http://www.osgi.org/

[8] New functionalities can be added to/removed from the backend system during runtime.

Evaluation: How We Tested and Optimized Elisa

Ricard Barberà-Guillem, Nadia Campos, Stephan Biel,
Martin Burkhard, Stefanie Erdt, Javier Ganzarain,
Gustavo Monleón, Andrea Nutsi and Ute Vidal Cabello

1 Executive Summary

During the different stages of the development process, it is necessary to introduce elements of evaluation to ensure that at the end of the process we will obtain a product covering the users' needs on a wide range of aspects such as functionality, accessibility or usability of the system as well as perception or willingness to purchase the product.

Three main stages of development were considered: contextualization, conceptualization and optimization. For each of these stages, this chapter details the validation techniques employed and the main results obtained. This includes, among others, the assessment of different concepts and mock-ups, as well as the validation of different prototypes under controlled conditions as well as in a real-use environment. Each evaluation contributed new input to ensure that, at the end of the innovation process, there would be more than just a suitable device for elderly people.

R. Barberà-Guillem (✉) · N. Campos
Instituto de Biomecánica de Valencia, Valencia, Spain
e-mail: ricard.barbera@ibv.upv.es

S. Biel · J. Ganzarain
Tioman & Partners SL, Barcelona, Spain

M. Burkhard · A. Nutsi
Universität der Bundeswehr München, Neubiberg, Germany

S. Erdt
Innovationsmanufaktur GmbH, Munich, Germany

G. Monleón
Servicios de Teleasistencia, Madrid, Spain

U. Vidal Cabello
VIOS Medien GmbH, Gröbenzell, Germany

E. F. Moritz (ed.), *Assistive Technologies for the Interaction of the Elderly*,
Advanced Technologies and Societal Change, DOI: 10.1007/978-3-319-00678-9_9,
© Springer International Publishing Switzerland 2014

2 Main Results

The evaluation process produced various results. The first and most direct one was the development of tools and methodologies adapted to the elderly. The second was that the different evaluations of the system were used as new input for the subsequent steps in the innovation process. In addition, the evaluations were a key element in comparing different alternatives, for instance the supporting hardware, as well as for the validation of hypotheses by the development team or the support of new ones (for instance in relation to the business model).

In summary, the evaluation continuously accompanied the innovation process, enabling us to confirm our initial profiles of the elderly and to obtain a positive overall evaluation of the product. Finally, we identified aspects the elderly regarded as vital to consider for the market introduction.

From a conceptual point of view, a development process can be divided into three main stages: contextualization, conceptualization and development. These phases cover at least a first identification of needs, the development of first concepts and the manufacturing of different prototypes. Table 1 summarizes the main elements evaluated and the results obtained in each of these steps. Each evaluation activity is a required step in the path to optimization, starting with the initial ideas and finishing with the final product, progressing through different intermediate prototypes. However, it is not just a straightforward process because several iterations and loops are required.

3 Storyline

User Involvement: How We Integrated Users into the Innovation Process and What We Learned from it already focused on "how" and "when" users could be integrated in the process of development, sometimes as providers of needs and desires but also as necessary evaluators of the proposed designs and functionalities. This chapter will instead focus more on "why" and "what" we had to validate and how the results obtained were integrated into the innovation process.

The main motivation for evaluating is to ensure a proper response, in each of the development phases, to the following specific questions:

1. In relation to the functionalities of the system

   - Does the system cope with the interests and needs of the user?
   - What can the user do with the system?
2. In relation to the accessibility and usability of the system

   - Can the user take advantage of the functionalities of the system?
   - Or is it too difficult to use or to understand?

Table 1 Summary of the validation process, main results and phase of development

Phase of development	Aspects and elements evaluated	Main results
Contextualization	Opening phase, no specific validation performed	Context and core functions common understanding
		Wide list of needs and demands of users
Conceptualization	Accessibility and usability (ISO 9241-9 2002)	Scenarios of use and personas
	#Prototype 0	Selection of hardware support
	Concept, acceptance, perception and purchase intention	Initial list of technical specifications
	#Prototype I	List of new requirements and recommendations to be improved/ implemented in prototype II
Development	Functionality	List of new requirements and recommendations to be improved/ implemented in prototype III
	Accessibility and usability	List of new requirements and recommendations to be improved/ implemented in the final product
	Concept, acceptance, perception and purchase intention	Identification of key elements of the market
	#Prototype II	
	#Prototype III	

3. In relation to the perception and purchase intention

- Does the system appeal to the user?
- Is the user willing to purchase the Elisa system?

The following describes the main results of the evaluation for each of the innovation phases as well as the more relevant aspects of the tools and methodologies used.

3.1 Evaluation During the Contextualization Phase

The objective of this phase was to obtain a broad vision of the problem and to really understand the context of communication, the use of ICT, and the key elements related to the socialization of the elderly population. To achieve this goal, we performed an extensive bibliographic review. Important input also came from the direct participation of the users during the focus groups and the online survey. These activities allowed us to understand the context, to identify the core functions of the system, and to obtain a global and comprehensive view of the different aspects related to Elisa, including as well a long list of demands and needs of the users.

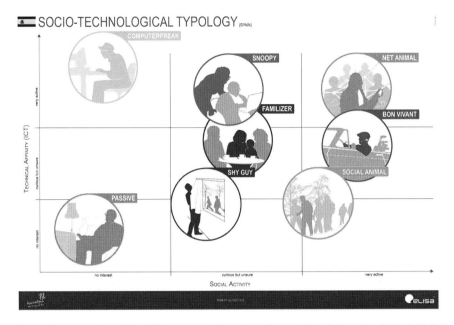

Fig. 1 Representation of the different types of users based on social activity and technical affinity

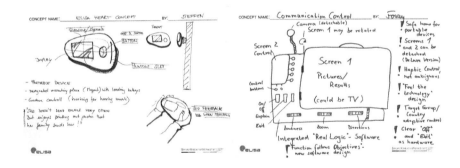

Fig. 2 Two different proposals for the hardware

One of the key activities in the contextualization phase was the identification of the different types of users, based on the social activity and the technical affinity. Figure 1 shows these typologies for the Spanish users, slightly different from the German ones. We constructed each type considering three main aspects: (1) personality, (2) social and leisure activities and (3) technical affinity.

During the contextualization phase we did not perform specific validation and assessment activities. However, this phase was necessary to complete the supporting background to develop the first concepts. Formally, this phase finished with an intensive creative concept finding workshop, in which, taking into account the different views of all partners, we defined the first concepts of the system. Figures 2 and 3

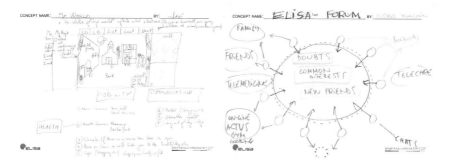

Fig. 3 Two different proposals for the interface/the network

Table 2 Description of the tablets and test parameters for ISO 92941-2

	Samsung galaxy tab 7.0TM	Samsung galaxy tab 10.1 NTM	Sony tablet STM	Sony tablet PTM
Display size (mm)	7.0″	10.1″	9.4″	2 × 5.5″
Screen resolution (width × height in pixels)	1024 × 600	1280 × 752	1280 × 752	1024 × 912
Pixel density (in DPI)	168.9	149.8	161.3	206.5
ISO D (in mm)	63.42	101.40	92.28	86.80
ISO W (in mm) for ISO ID (2.5/3.0/3.5/4.0)	13.53/9.02 6.01/4.21	21.70/14.41 9.83/6.61	19.84/13.07 8.82/6.14	18.62/12.33 8.38/5.67

D distance, *ID* index of difficulty, *W* width as defined in ISO 92941-2

show some of the ideas worked out during the workshop. While the concepts in Fig. 2 focus on the hardware, the concepts in Fig. 3 focus more on the interface and on the network behind the system.

3.2 Evaluation During the Conceptualization Phase

The objective of this phase was to define the first concepts while taking into account the defined context. One of the first challenges was organizing and prioritizing the information. The second was defining the key aspects of the future application including the supporting hardware.

From the bibliographic review and complementing analyses, it was quite clear that the best option to support the application was a tablet device; the trouble was selecting the right one. Thus, we performed a comparison test with four different devices (#prototype 0) using the methodology proposed by ISO 92941-2. Table 2 describes the characteristics of the four tablets assessed during the validation process (#prototype 0) and the main parameters of the ISO 92941-2 test (ISO 9241-9 2002).

Table 3 Recorded MDTT error rate of evaluators in Spain and Germany

Error rate of multi-directional tapping task			
Galaxy tab 7.0	Galaxy tab 10.1 N	Tablet S	Tablet P
Country			
Spain			
61.8 %	38.3 %	47.5 %	46.9 %
(SD = 44.11)	(SD = 9.01)	(SD = 21.18)	(SD = 24,91)
Germany			
50.1 %	36.8 %	43.1 %	41.6 %
(SD = 24.27)	(SD = 7.17)	(SD = 15.17)	(SD = 14.45)
Total			
55.9 %	37.6 %	45.3 %	44.2 %
(SD = 35.99)	(SD = 8.01)	(SD = 18.81)	(SD = 20.58)

SD standard deviation

Table 4 Tablet rankings based on placements by interviewees in Spain and Germany

Tablet ranking			
Galaxy tab 7.0	Galaxy tab 10.1 N	Tablet S	Tablet P
Country			
Spain			
3rd place (32)	2nd place (38)	1st place (42)	2nd place (38)
Germany			
2nd place (37)	1st place (44)	4th place (34)	3rd place (35)
Total			
4th place (69)	1st place (82)	2nd place (76)	3rd place (73)

4-points ranking: 1st place = 4 points, 2nd place = 3 points, 3rd place = 2 points, 4th place = 1 point

Thirty users participated in this validation. We recorded the error rate of the multi-directional tapping task (Table 2) and the ranking given by the users to the tablets after completing all tests (Table 3) (Burkhard and Koch 2012). The ranking given by the users was coherent with the error values for the best and worst cases (Table 4). Finally, we selected the Galaxy tab 10.1 N as the hardware to implement Elisa on.

Also in the contextualization phase, we developed two different GUI approaches to a state of mock-ups (Fig. 4). One was defined as content-centric and the other as person-centric (#prototype I). With these mock-ups, we evaluated the concept, acceptance, perception and purchase intention.

Users perceived the two GUI proposals, content- and person-centric, as being markedly different. Some preferred the content- and others the person-centric GUI. However, in both cases they missed the parts that were not available in their preferred GUI: The ones who liked the content-centric approach missed a more direct contact with their friends, while the ones who liked the person-centric missed direct links to main interests or contents.

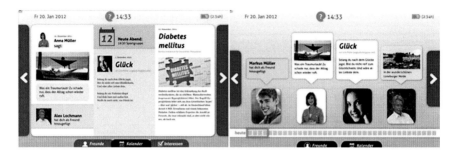

Fig. 4 Content-centric (*left*) and person-centric (*right*) start screen interface

Other important results from this phase were the construction of the use scenarios and of the personas, the selection of the hardware in which the Elisa system was to be implemented, as well as a more detailed list of technical specifications and recommendations to be implemented in prototype II, for instance the best aspects of the two GUI approaches.

3.3 Evaluation During the Development Phase

We defined this phase as beginning with the first functional prototype (#prototype II) and ending with the development of recommendations to be implemented in the final product. At the beginning of this phase, we had a clear idea of the concept we wanted to develop, including the GUI proposal, the supporting hardware and the underlying middleware necessary to make life easier for the end user. The challenge in this case was further developing the functional prototype (#prototype II) into the final product, that is, a real environment use prototype (#prototype III), as completely as possible.

Figure 5 shows an example of the results obtained with the SIMPLIT methodology (Durá et al. 2012) during the validation of the usability aspects of the interface for prototype II. Despite the generally good results, there still were improvement recommendations for the developers of the Elisa system.

Figure 6 shows the final location for the arrow buttons and the tabs. This location was validated by experts of the consortium involved in the usability tests and by users. Following the results of the validation, we decided to put the tabs on the bottom (better ergonomics and readability) and put the arrow buttons back on both sides (more natural placement).

As we got closer to the final prototype, it became increasingly important to check the components relative to the market, such as purchase intention or the appeal of the product. Tables 5 and 6 show information obtained directly from the users during the validation process. This information needed to be taken into consideration for the definition of the go-to-market strategies.

TASK 1. "User identification"

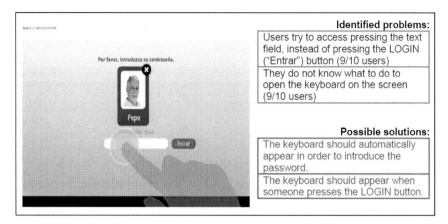

Fig. 5 Example of a result of the validation by the SIMPLIT methodology

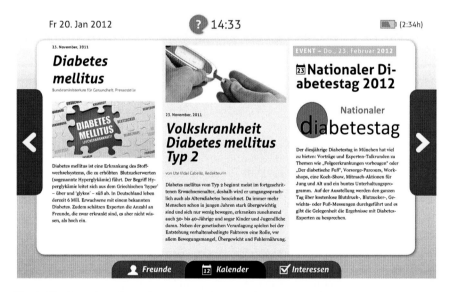

Fig. 6 Final location of the tabs and arrow buttons after the validation results

The validation of prototype III was the most difficult and challenging because the users took the Elisa system to their homes and had to perform different tasks autonomously. During the kick off meeting for this validation, users met the technical team; especially important was the direct contact to the person on the Elisa hotline to simplify future interactions. During this session, each of the participants in the validation received a personalized tablet with the Elisa software,

Table 5 Main aspects of Elisa purchase considering different user typologies

	Typology					
	Snoopy	Bon Vivant	Familizer	Shy Guy	Social Animal	Super User
Do you like the look and feel of Elisa?	Yes		Not too much		Yes	
Elisa perception	*Interesting and practical*					
Places where users buy electronic devices	Electronics market		Local telecommunication shop			
Places where users would buy Elisa	Electronics market		Specialist supplier/ local shop			
Rang of price (max.)	500 €		700 €		500 €	
Support on the use of electronic devices	*Relatives*					
Sources of information on electronic devices	*Friends/relatives*					
Purchase intention	Yes		Yes	Yes	Not sure	No

Note Empty cells mean that non-determinant conclusions were obtained

Table 6 Highest scored place/s to buy the Elisa device for each country

	Country	
	Germany	Spain
Places where users buy electronic devices	Specialists suppliers/local shops	Local telecommunication shop
Places where users would buy Elisa	Specialists suppliers/local shops	Electronics market/generalist retailer
Range of price (max.)	500 €	750 €
Service contract		Yes
Support on the use of electronic devices	Relatives/friends	Experts/relatives
Sources of information on electronic devices	Magazines/internet	Friends/relatives/internet
Purchase intention	Yes	Yes

Note Empty cells mean that non-determinant conclusions were obtained

the test handbook and the evaluation sheets for each of the tasks they had to perform. Table 7 shows the tasks for the first week for Germany; in Spain, the tasks were slightly different. During the second week, the users could use the Elisa tablets at will.

Table 8 shows the main characteristics of the twenty users participating in the validation in a real use environment.

As regards especially the users with low-tech profiles, they were very pleased to be able to use a technical gadget by themselves and have the possibility to be in touch with their friends and families. They also liked the possibility of finding

Table 7 Tasks the users had to perform during the first week of test

Day	Task 1	Task 2	Task 3
1	Watch the three Elisa tutorials	Answer the welcome message from TP 55	Look at the articles in the interest section and read one article
2	Read one activity	Add an activity to your personal activities	Call the Elisa Skype hotline
3	Read and recommend one article	Adapt personal interests	Look for test users with similar hobbies
4	Invite someone to an activity	Send a message	Activate all categories in interests
5	Look at personal activities	Answer the message from the "Treffpunkt 55plus" magazine	Call someone via Skype
6	Send a message concerning your activity invitation Check if the person receives your invitation	Adapt the activities to your personal interests	Read and recommend one article
7	Send a message	Activate all categories in activities	Add an activity to your personal activities

Table 8 Main data of the users participating in the last validation

	Total	Germany	Spain
Number of participants	20	10	10
Gender	13 women (65 %)	7 women (70 %)	6 women (60 %)
	7 men (35 %)	3 men (30 %)	4 men (40 %)
Types	5 Snoopy	3 Snoopy	2 Snoopy
	4 Bon Vivant	2 Bon Vivant	2 Bon Vivant
	4 Familizer	2 Familizer	2 Familizer
	4 Shy Guy	2 Shy Guy	2 Shy Guy
	3 Social Animal	1 Social Animal	2 Social Animal

people with similar interests. They consider the Elisa system a good starting point for using IT tools. Elisa actually represents a breakthrough for them.

Some of the demands for new functionalities to be added, especially from the advanced users, were the possibility to have Elisa in a computer or laptop version as well, free browser, games and "funny things" and online ticket sales/reservation. The calendar was another part the users felt could be improved to make it more intuitive to use and, specifically, to be able to add new activities by themselves.

Focusing on accessibility and usability of the system, the keyboard received negative attention from the users, even from the ones with a high tech profile.

Users also complained about some of the expressions used in the interface, as they had problems understanding them.

As a conclusion, we can however say that elderly people showed great interest in Elisa and were willing to buy it and use it.

References

Burkhard, M., Koch, M.: Evaluating touchscreen interfaces of tablet computers for elderly people. In: Reiterer, H., Deussen, O. (eds.) Mensch & Computer 2012—Workshopband: interaktiv informiert—allgegenwärtig und allumfassend!?, pp. 33–59. Oldenbourg Verlag, München (2012)

Durá, J.V, Laparra, J., Poveda, R., Marzo, R., López, A., Bollaín, C.: SIMPLIT: Ensuring technology usability for the elderly. Gerontechnology **11**(2) (2012). http://gerontechnology. info/index.php/journal/article/view/gt.2012.11.02.279.00/1645

ISO 9241-9: Evaluating Non-Keyboard Input Devices (2002)

Business: How We Worked to Get Elisa into the Market and Share the Benefits

Wilhelm Prasser and Fee Wiebusch

1 Executive Summary

This chapter explains how we established a business plan for Elisa. After first analyzing the market, that is, the wants of the elderly as well as already existing products, we then examined different business models. After choosing one, we developed a whole business plan and started talks with investors.

2 Main Results

At the very beginning of the project we simply agreed on one major goal—to bring the product to the market. A common denominator between all the involved parties was "we are only successful if we see our product in some retail shops where the elderly can buy it". So each step we took and each decision we made was designed to bring us one step closer to our goal. Under this proposition we structured our approach for the go-to-market.

> Business Model: Several Ways to Launch Elisa

After a closer look at the results of the market analysis we started thinking about possible business models, thus preparing a framework in which the created value, the necessary resources and the appropriate sales channels match the needs

W. Prasser (✉)
Data United GmbH, Munich, Germany
e-mail: wilhelm.prasser@data-united.de

F. Wiebusch
Brainware GmbH, Stuttgart, Germany

E. F. Moritz (ed.), *Assistive Technologies for the Interaction of the Elderly*,
Advanced Technologies and Societal Change, DOI: 10.1007/978-3-319-00678-9_10,
© Springer International Publishing Switzerland 2014

of the target audience. In several brainstorming and business sessions, we developed a well-structured approach which at first glance may seem a bit old-fashioned but taking into account the experience we gained and the future ideas we have, it was a quite reasonable starting point.

> Investors' Talk: Coming Up with the Money

As soon as the aforementioned "big boys" will have been targeted, they need to be wowed. We think the combination of a tremendously big customer base and an already proven market approach (for example Facebook.com—even though we do have a different client group) gives us substantial momentum in the arena of investments.

Let's start with the first step we took—the market analysis and its findings.

3 Storyline

3.1 Business Model: Several Ways to Launch Elisa

We developed the business model in a very classic way combined with a step-by-step approach with the consortium partners and the end user. However, the go-to-market (G2M) approach was somehow different with our Lean StartUp strategy as a first step into the market.

The general approach to the business model was using a holistic model to define a stable and robust business model, including an appropriate value chain and some advice for possible next steps. We proceeded as follows:

- Definition of one valid business model out of three proven possibilities
- Definition of the value chain according to the business model
- Provision of input for the business planning.

3.1.1 General Approach

To align the business model with the general approach within the SI-Screen/Elisa project, the consortium agreed to a so-called step-by-step model to achieve the best results for the business model design. The steps we took towards the design, the validation and the implementation of the business model and its value chain were:

- Definition of one valid business model out of three proven possibilities
- Validation of this business model with end users, business partners (along the value chain) and the involved partners within the consortium

- Based on the validation in step two, adaptation and redesign of parts of the business model (feedback mechanism).

There are several ways to develop a proper business model and there are also a lot of different business models already described and implemented today. The questions that have to be addressed are:

- What are the most relevant business models for Elisa?
- How do they fit into the big picture as we move from the business model and the value chain to an overall business plan?
- What are the steps to be taken to guarantee a successful launch of Elisa in different markets?

After a closer look at all the possibilities, we found that there were several models which fit the overall approach. Appropriate business models we considered in greater detail were:

- The Distribution Business Model via channels: classic offline business model (retail)—this business model has already been existing for years and is the classic way to approach clients via well-known channels.
- The Bricks and Clicks Business Model: online business model (AppStore)—an additional business model mainly driven by Apple's go-to-market approach. Elisa clients may not adopt this concept immediately but the possibility of taking that direction will be quite relevant in the mid-term.
- The Network Effects Business Model (Wikinomics)—a new approach of generating business in the Web 2.0 which allows business partners to cooperate in a flexible way, build up businesses on the fly and market demands. In terms of SI-Screen/Elisa, this model allows a flexible adaption to future business concepts and market segments not addressed in the present.

3.1.2 Business Model Canvas

To reconcile all the above-mentioned topics and make them more comprehensive, the so-called Business Model Canvas is an excellent framework to work with. It shows how the different areas are positioned along the business model and what the topics to be addressed are. The Business Model Canvas is quite a good way to describe the different areas important to designing a robust and comprehensive business model. It also shows how the different areas are linked to each other. After having filled the different areas with relevant content, we allocated the single sectors to partners we saw as major players in those areas to achieve a successful launch (Fig. 1).

Figure 2 shows how the different areas will work together and how certain functionalities and tasks are performed—internally and externally.

To combine everything into a robust business model, we summarized and compared the three different possible business models as shown in Table 1. The most simple of these models is the so-called retail model, which is well established

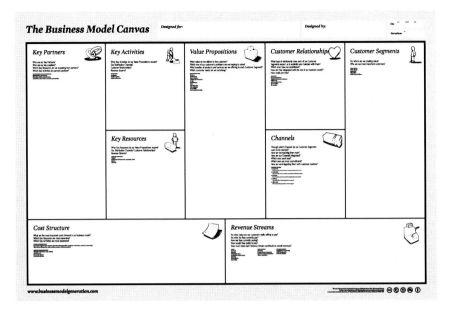

Fig. 1 Business model canvas based on Osterwalder and Pigneur (2010)

and has been proven in several areas. The most advanced business model in the 2.0 world is the Wikinomics Business Model. In this model, different parts or modules of the solution are available in an open source world and could be combined and performed quite flexibly. On the other hand, the revenue sharing in this model is based on the performance and the provided task.

3.1.3 Decision Making: Business Model Retail

This business model describes the "classic" way for the go-to-market (G2M) approach. We decided to pursue this direction after analyzing all the pros and cons because it fits the concept paper developed earlier quite well. The approach is to develop an application for a tablet computer, which replaces the standard graphical user interface (GUI) with the Elisa GUI.

3.1.4 The Appropriate Value Chain

The value chain of Elisa is the chain of activities which are processed to address the specific needs of (the value for) the target market. Elisa passes through all stages of the chain and at each stage, the product gains some additional value.

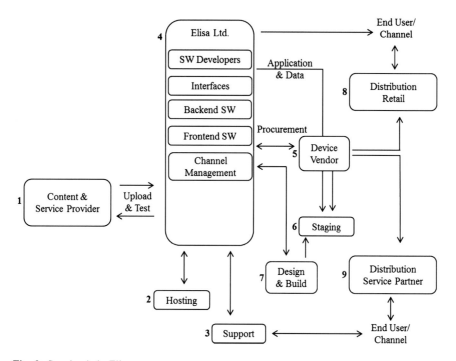

Fig. 2 Supply chain Elisa

Table 1 Three business models

	Retail	Online	Wikinomics
Well-known	X	X	–
Defined processes	X	X	–
Easy roll-out	X	X	–
Central/distributed	Central	Central	Distributed
Clear roles and responsibilities	X	X	–
Branding	X	X	–
Market coverage	X (cost)	X (access)	X
Flexibility	–	X/–	X
Add-on features	–	–	X
Scalability	–	X	X

The value-chain concept has been extended beyond the Elisa core development. It will apply to the whole supply chain and distribution networks. The delivery of our product and services to the end customer will mobilize different economic factors, each managing its own value chain.

- Inbound logistics

  – Information and content supply chain
  – Device vendors
  – OS platforms (operating system)
  – Connectivity of partners (data exchange)

- Operations

  – Product development
  – Design and customization
  – Integration (interfaces for content and services)

- Outbound logistics

  – Distribution
  – Original equipment manufacturer (OEM)
  – Consulting

- Marketing and sales

  – G2M (go to market)
  – CRM (customer relationship management)
  – Partner programs (affiliate, funding etc.)

- Service

  – Support and helpdesk
  – Maintenance
  – Online avatar
  – Self-healing functionalities

- Technology (R&D)

  – Backend system
  – Frontend system
  – Communication.

The major value that needs to be provided by the different areas in the value chain is

- Relevance—by proven content and services
- Easiness—by adaptive interface and a dedicated G2M
- Security—by user data protection
- Reliability—by a seamless support concept.

The advantage of the Elisa platform is not only the advanced GUI but also the possibility to design and align the content and the functionalities along the value chain (internal and external) to the market needs or user demands. The deliverables and functionalities (services and content) of the platform can easily be tailored to local (geographical) needs, so that different requirements can be implemented flexibly.

Table 2 Market requirements

Business model	Value provided
Retail (distribution)	Trusted sales channel
	Easy to buy
	Seamless support structure
Product (design)	All in one
	Easy to use
	No technologic hassle
Go-to-market (G2M)	Integrated approach (channel & Elisa Ltd)
	Feedback loops
	Target market focus
Supply chain	Relevant content and services
	Device vendor-independent
	Focus on core competencies (Elisa Ltd, service provider, supplier)

3.1.5 Summary of the Business Model and Value Chain: Design, Build and Operate the Window of Social Interaction for the Elderly

Table 2 addresses the basic assumptions for a successful business plan and also the general market requirements for a state-of-the-art product.

3.2 Investors' Talk: Coming Up with the Money

The best way to draw the attention of the "guys with the money" is to create a story that awakens their interest. This was the first step of our investor presentation: telling the story of "Facebook for the elderly" (and big dollar signs appeared in their eyes due to Facebook's big success) and giving them an idea about the market (70 million potential users in the EU alone).

Looking into the entire solution, it becomes quite obvious that there already are several major players along the value chain and within the business model. These key players could—or so we thought—also act as potential investors because the success of our solution brings them closer to potential users and they are already involved in the go-to-market. The key players we addressed were:

- Telecommunications companies (telcos)
- Institutional investors
- Business angels.

Institutional investors usually do not invest in start-ups (seed funding) as they want to see a reliable pre-existing revenue stream. Telcos on the other hand are very interested in attracting new customers, because their competition is quite tough and Elisa could easily bring them a million new users. Business Angels are also quite interested, but you typically need more than one so the investment can be split between them and that requires a lot of time-consuming coordination.

To cut a long story short, at the time of writing we are in talks with several different investors and have hopes of finding the perfect match soon.

Questions we were prepared to answer during our pitch were:

- Market size
- Market capitalization
- Already existing solutions—SWOT analysis
- Revenue models
- IPR.

All in all, we came full circle from the market analysis all the way to the business plan and investor presentation. The last step to full success that at the time of writing still needed to be completed is the go-to-market phase for which we are, however, dependent on feedback from the investors. Our work is only done if we can launch Elisa and make it available to its intended users—which brings us back to the beginning of this chapter: Success means that the elderly can (and will) buy Elisa.

Reference

Osterwalder, A., Pigneur, Y.: Business Model Generation. Ein Handbuch für Visionäre, Spielveränderer und Herausforderer. Campus Verlag GmbH, Frankfurt am Main (2010)

Product: What We Generated in this Project

Javier Gámez Payá

1 Executive Summary

We are almost at the end of this book, after the description of the process, the target group, and the methodology of the validation, among other; it is now time to describe what the product Elisa actually is, that is, what defines the final outcome of the project that we intend to bring to the market.

Elisa will not be successful due to its separate parts. Rather, it is its combination of different parts that makes it innovative and unique in the market.

In this chapter, we are thus going to present all the parts, components, pieces that make up Elisa. It should be pointed out, however, that due to the content and objective of this chapter, we are only going to present the main results and not the storyline and scientific excursion as we did in the previous chapters.

2 Main Results

Generally seen, Elisa is a window and an access door to a great number of possibilities to improve the quality of life of the elderly generation. It is a powerful social interaction tool that improves social inclusion and avoids social isolation, enabling the elderly to stay in contact with their relatives and friends, to get to know new friends, to enroll in new and inspiring activities, as well as to be informed about interesting topics. It should be pointed out that nowadays, elderly social isolation is one of the main problems Europe is facing.

The success of Elisa is based on a well-thought-out combination of software and hardware features, and thus we can say with conviction that the whole is more than the sum of its parts. Its development is based on the participation of elderly

J. Gámez Payá (✉)
Innovationsmanufaktur GmbH, Munich, Germany
e-mail: jgp@innovationsmanufaktur.com

E. F. Moritz (ed.), *Assistive Technologies for the Interaction of the Elderly*,
Advanced Technologies and Societal Change, DOI: 10.1007/978-3-319-00678-9_11,
© Springer International Publishing Switzerland 2014

users, from the early beginning, that helped to obtain the SIMPLIT label, a seal of approval, which certifies that a product is comfortable, intuitive and easy to use guaranteeing that the products consider the needs, preferences and special characteristics of elderly people.[1] In detail Elisa consists of (Fig. 1):

- A **software** that has three parts:

    (1) Backend system—Social Software Integration Layer (SSIL)
    (2) Frontend system—Graphical user interface (GUI)
    (3) User application in a mobile device—Android application

- **Hardware** that consists of a leather housing frame and a stand to increase usability

The Elisa system's unique selling propositions (USPs) are:

- Functioning prototype tested in successive instances of user involvement
- Intuitive, friendly and easy-to-use GUI
- Filtered and reliable content for the elderly
- Successful vision and a passionate team for further developments
- Hardware model by Porsche Design Studio
- Flexible and open source backend system

Backend system—the Social Software Integration Layer
The backend system of Elisa has been explained in detail in Chap. Social Software Integration: How We Integrated Different Interaction Features and Technologies of this book. However, I am going to shortly summarize its main functions that make it unique and special, what kind of content we provide, as well as the principal features that differentiate it from the competition.

Functions of the SSIL:

- To gather information from the internet adapted to the end users' needs
- To give and facilitate the access to different social network services (SNS)
- To synchronize with other SNS
- To filter the more relevant information regarding the user's personal preferences to avoid overwhelming elderly people
- To organize and show the information gathered in an easy, comprehensive, friendly and consistent way

Content of the SSIL:
To decide on the main sections and the information included in Elisa, we organized several focus groups, interviews and surveys to ask the end users about their preferences and needs. As a result of those studies we decided to structure the content into three sections (see Table 1):

---

[1] Detailed information about the SIMPLIT seal and methodology is available on the official site http://www.simplit.es/ in English, Spanish and Portuguese.

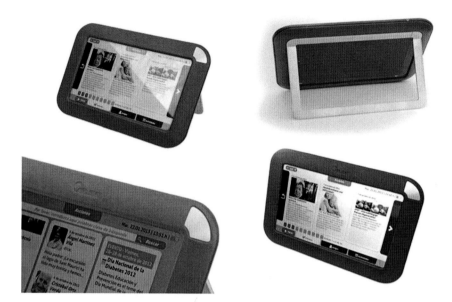

Fig. 1 Elisa at a glance

Table 1 Elisa sections

Section	Objective
Friends	Enhance social communication
	Improve existing relationships
	Generate new relationships
	Promote the social interaction among elderly people
Interests	Inform about interesting topics
	Provide trustable information of topics related to: health, leisure, travel, culture, learning…
	Motivate elderly people to read and learn something new
	Promote the exchange of knowledge and information among elderly people
Activities	Inspire elderly people to do something new and challenging
	Motivate elderly people to enroll in leisure and wellbeing activities in their vicinity
	Promote the social interaction among elderly people

Regarding the features of the system, we can point out three that make the SSIL unique:

- The SSIL is able to preserve the privacy of personal data of the end user.
- Elisa users are relived from administrative tasks such as account registration or social network management required by other SNS: Administrative tasks can be delegated to a person of trust.

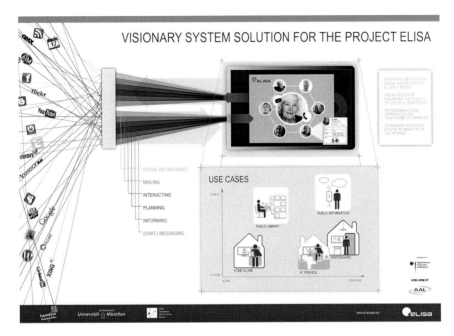

Fig. 2 Social software integration layer

- The SSIL unifies the content of all existing SNS (Facebook, Google+...), web feeds, contact management systems, social content sharing platforms, and so on in one single information stream that will give the elderly the impression of taking part in only one homogeneous community.

Figure 2 depicts how the SSIL works. On the left side, we see all the information and contents from the SNS, then, as seen in the middle, the SSIL gathers, organizes, filters and finally shows the information to the end user and on the right side, we see how the end user's input goes back into the SNS. At the bottom on the right, we can see several examples of use cases of the system. Since this is a portable system it can be used at home or outdoors, alone or in company.

Graphical user interface

The GUI we developed for Elisa offers a new way to interact with technological devices such as tablet PCs. The end users that participated in the prototype evaluation claimed that the usage of Elisa is very challenging and enjoyable at the same time. Moreover, the look and feel of Elisa represents an improvement over the typical and complicated GUI that we are used to in current SNS.

The main features of the Elisa GUI are presented in detail in User Interface Design; however, I am going to sum up the main ones that altogether make our proposal unique and cutting-edge (Table 2).

As already mentioned, the content of Elisa is split into three sections. Next, we are going to present the main screen and those three sections. Regarding the main

Table 2 Graphical user interface features

Feature	Remark
Usability	Intuitive and easy-to-use system with a smooth learning curve
	The Elisa UI shows Facebook/Google+ posts, photos, e-mails, shared articles all in the same look-and-feel. The user can read and reply to messages without needing to care about the communication channel
	The main screen shows the most recent activities from people on the contact list in inverse chronological order
	The so-called cards concept: content and interactive elements are consistently presented inside rectangular frames, which are easier to use than the conventional WIMP (window, Icon, Mouse, Pointer) paradigm
Ergonomics	Adapted to finger movement and anthropometrics
	Adapted to the use condition of the device (on the table or hand-held)
Navigation	Horizontal navigation concept that makes it very easy to follow the navigation process, thus, the user is aware of where he/she is at every moment
	Two ways to navigate: using the arrow bottoms that are very intuitive or through the use of swipe gestures
Look-and-feel	"Friendly" design
	Size similar to an open book
Adapted user interface	User's technical experience is taken into consideration, and only simple functionalities are offered for beginners. Based on the users' behavior, the Elisa UI will gradually unlock functionalities as the user becomes familiar with the existing functionality
	The user is able to choose which activities he/she is interested in, so the system will display him/her only information on the selected activities
Animation	Carefully designed speed in order to be neither too fast nor too slow, so the end user is now able to easily follow the horizontal navigation concept

screen, we used the card concept to show Elisa information (interests, friends and activities). The newest messages, feeds, or activities are displayed in summaries; the user can read the details by tapping on them (Fig. 3).

In the interests section, the end user can find the so-called Elisa magazine that consists of a great number of hot topic articles from trustable sources, that is, written by professionals such as doctors, engineers, or health care professionals. In order to structure the overall content, for the time being we divided the articles into five categories:

- Health and social wellbeing
- Culture
- Travelling
- Society
- Living and care

The user can choose his or her topics of interest, thus adapting the Elisa content to the individual user's preferences, likes and dislikes. Once the interests section is opened, all the articles are displayed following the card concept. Each card consists of a picture and an abstract; if one is selected, the whole article can be read

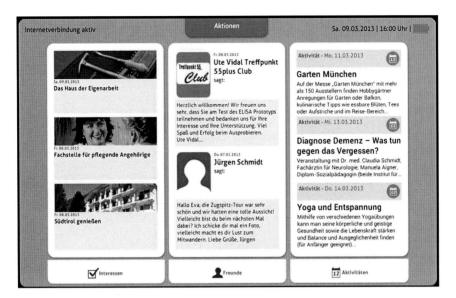

Fig. 3 Elisa main screen

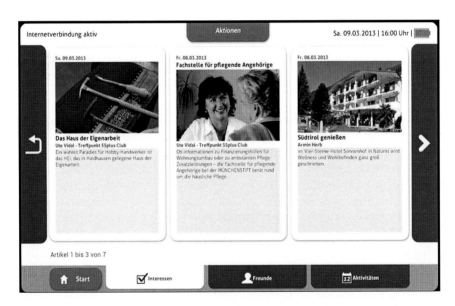

Fig. 4 Interests section

(Fig. 4). Once read, the article can easily be sent and recommended to a friend; the objective behind this is to promote social relationships and the exchange of valuable information.

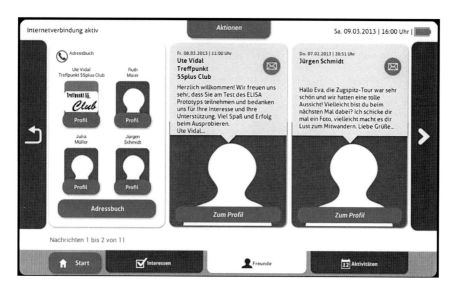

Fig. 5 Friends section

If the friends section is selected, the users can see their family and friends and their contact details. Moreover, Elisa costumers will be able to send messages, perform voice calls and video calls, as well as send invitations to events and activities. Equally, Elisa users can receive messages and invitations from their contact persons (Fig. 5).

In the activity section, Elisa users are able to see all the activities happening around them. If the user taps on one activity, he/she can learn more details about it such as: when, where, how long … Moreover, the application also enables them to send invitations to other friends (Fig. 6). It should be highlighted that in this section as well, the user is able to choose from five categories of activities:

- Health and fitness
- Culture
- Trips and guided tours
- Workshops and classes
- My city

User application in a mobile device—Android App

After the development of the backend and frontend system, our further aim was to spread Elisa utilizing as many different devices as possible. Thus, the best choice for us was to develop a mobile application using the Android Operating System (OS). There are three main reasons why we opted for this OS:

- It had approximately 70 % of the market share in 2013.
- There are many companies that use this OS, for example Sony, LG, HTC, Lenovo, among others.
- It is an open source OS.

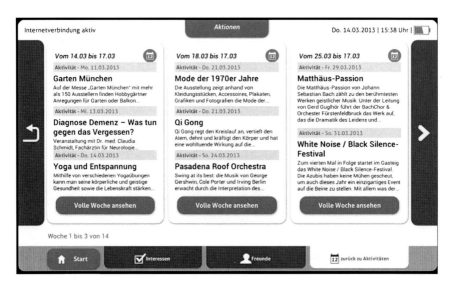

Fig. 6 Activities section

Table 3 Hardware target features and design solutions

Feature	Design solution
High usability	Adapted frame to the hands of the elderly considering the ergonomic and usability principles (Fig. 7)
Better feeling	A frame made out of high quality leather (Fig. 8)
Uniqueness	First leather frame in the market (Fig. 8)
High screen protection	The frame design protects the screen in case the user accidentally places the tablet PC face down (Fig. 9)
Usage condition improvement	The frame has a stand on the back so the user can put it on a table very easily (Fig. 10)

It should be highlighted that, since the backend and frontend systems are independent from the user application (for now Android App), in the future we are going to be able to develop new applications compatible with other OS such as iOS and Windows, thus covering almost 100 % of the tablets market.

Hardware

During our research we encountered several problems that elderly people have with current tablet housings; some of them apply to other target groups as well:

- Elderly people are afraid to crash their tablet, due its weak look-and-feel.
- All tablet PCs are made out of plastic or metal, and thus have the appearance of just another high tech product that is not user-friendly for non-tech people.
- Elderly people have difficulties holding the current tablets due to their thin frames.

Fig. 7 Ergonomic frame design

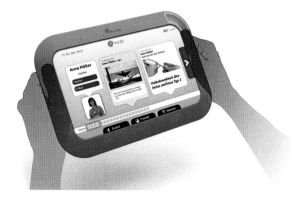

Fig. 8 Frame material: leather

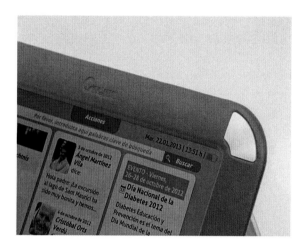

Fig. 9 Screen protection

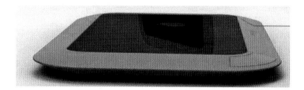

- Current tablets do not provide any protection for the screen; once again, the consumer is supposed to buy a protective sleeve to keep the screen in a good state.

All the above aspects led us to propose a new element complementing the current hardware, that is, a new housing design. Table 3 shows the target features and the design solution for every one of them.

Fig. 10 Elisa stand design

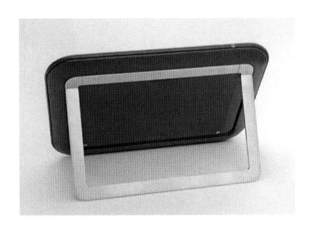

3 Next Stop, the Market

Currently, we have a high quality prototype ready to start the go-to-market phase. In order to achieve this final goal we are now

- Improving the design and consistency of our prototype in order to turn it into a final product for the market.
- Seeking investors who will help us to bring it to the market in several European countries.

Recommendations: What We Suggest

Javier Gámez Payá, Stefanie Erdt and Eckehard Fozzy Moritz

1 Executive Summary

In this chapter we aim to share some recommendations and lessons that we have learnt during this project. They will be very helpful in similar projects; to avoid problems and mistakes, to progress faster, and to increase the relevance and success of future AAL projects.

We split the main recommendations into the following sections:

- Team composition
- Process definition
- Project work
- Reporting
- User integration
- Product focus
- Market introduction

2 Our Recommendations

There are three cornerstones in project management that should be considered in the roadmap of every single project; the recommendations shown below are aligned with them.

The first cornerstone is to keep the team motivated, so we present some recommendations that should be considered in the team composition of a project. The second one is to achieve a good project result, for which we propose some advice concerning the entire process definition, the daily work of the project, end user integration, product focus strategy, and market introduction. The third one is to

J. Gámez Payá (✉) · S. Erdt · E. F. Moritz
Innovationsmanufaktur GmbH, Munich, Germany
e-mail: jgp@innovationsmanufaktur.com

E. F. Moritz (ed.), *Assistive Technologies for the Interaction of the Elderly*,
Advanced Technologies and Societal Change, DOI: 10.1007/978-3-319-00678-9_12,
© Springer International Publishing Switzerland 2014

keep the sponsors happy, hence we share some recommendations related to the project reporting and the relationship between the team members and the sponsors.

Team composition

- Diversity of the team composition: The team should be heterogeneous with high social and professional competence. Social skills in a working team such as empathy, assertiveness or fluent communication are essential to achieving a good progress and to provide an enjoyable experience to all team members.
- Project motivation over the whole project duration: A motivated team is one of the key elements of a successful project. To achieve this, every participant in the project should identify with the task and the team, appreciate her/his own role, and gain external appreciation.
- Personality is more important than an institution (this may be difficult to take care of in a funded project, because you often cannot decide who will work in your project): This is once again related to the social skills of the group; whenever possible it is desirable to be able to choose the people that you want to work with.
- The whole value chain should be involved: This should be already considered in the preparation phase of the project; the proposal coordinator should make sure that the whole value chain is included in the project. However, the value chain does not necessarily stay the same over the whole course of the project; one should be ready for possible changes in the market that lead to changes in the value chain.
- Avoid changes in the team composition: These changes will cause

    - Loss of time, because the new member needs to catch up on the work done by his/her predecessor.
    - Loss of information and deep knowledge of the project development. It is very difficult to transfer all the information to the new team member, even in the best conditions.
    - Loss of work efficiency. New team members need to learn the working pace of the group and how to fit into it, and at the same time, the group has to become acquainted with how the new people work.
    - Loss of social awareness. New people in the group have to get to know the other team members in a social perspective as well.

Process definition

- Orientation according to a suitable Holistic Innovation process: In the case of this project, the process of Holistic Innovation (Moritz 2009) seemed best suited, as it combines systematic procedure with systemic thinking and is thus ideal for a complex, still undefined system development. However, in other projects other approaches may be superior.
- High importance of the preparatory phase before deciding on a concept: In accordance with Holistic Innovation processes, it is very important to consider and analyze the innovation context system and the functionalities to be realized

during the preparatory phase. This includes the characterization of end users, the understanding of their predispositions, motivations and barriers, trends and developments in relevant technologies, services and activities, use scenarios, stakeholders and many other dimensions.

- Switching from research (preparatory work) to the real development: During the first stages of the project, one often has to gather scientific and technical information on the current state of the art and other context issues. However, once this task is finished, one should focus on the development of the product that shall reach the market. As this means a radical change in orientation and working style, this is not an easy shift and needs to be well addressed by the project moderators.
- Internal communication of the process: Everybody must be aware what she/he is doing and why. As usually not everyone works according to the same process, the communication of those processes must not be omitted. This is all the more important if you apply new processes.
- Consequent orientation towards the process plan: It is very important to set a process plan and follow it. If one is forced to change it, this should be explained, possibly negotiated and reported to all team members as soon as possible.
- Appropriate forms and amount of end user integration: This is especially relevant in the first stages of the project and during the validation and evaluation of the prototype development. Proper end user integration will guarantee that the product meets consumer needs and has success in the market.
- Constant reviewing of the technological advancements and tech trends: In the course of the project, some technological advances might appear and might change either the technological development of the project, the business approach or how consumers will use the final product.

Project work

- Simple and effective project management, cooperation, and communication tools: As we learned the hard way, one should avoid using a complex strategy and realization of project management tools, as they often create a working burden in themselves rather than contributing to the project progress. In our case, mailing lists, a file sharing system, bilateral and group calls as well as meetings turned out to be most effective, plus a deliverables and timeline management.
- Clear guidelines by the project leader: It is the responsibility of the project and the work package leaders to give instructions and guidelines that are clear, consistent and widespread among the team.
- Regular personal contact: Phone calls, teleconferences and emails are very good communication tools; however, a personal touch is vital to achieving a high team spirit and good results in the project. Thus, a minimum of two personal meetings per year should be incorporated in the project schedule, all allowing for social activities as well.
- Social elements (team building) during project meetings: These activities are essential for any project. They

- improve the communication flow among team members,
- help to overcome social barriers and improve social relationships among team members (especially important in EU projects with different cultures and working styles),
- increase the identification with the project,
- generate a positive energy and atmosphere in the team.

Reporting

- Knowing the expectations of the sponsors: Funded projects have special obligations that must be considered. Much more than only focusing on a good project result, it is important to: (1) submit all reports and deliverables in time and (2) achieve the milestones proposed in the description of the work of the project. Furthermore, a good communication flow with the officials of the project is recommended.
- Meeting the deadlines: Since there will always be unexpected issues that can delay some tasks, a buffer should be included in the project plan to make sure that the deadlines can be met.
- Easy-to-use and clear templates and instructions: At the beginning of the project report, templates should be proposed with a clear structure that will remain consistent during the whole project. This will make it easier to produce and read the reports and present them to the reviewers for the project follow-up.
- Open communication with sponsors and national contact persons: Whenever possible one should meet with the sponsors in person, and if this is not possible at least try to organize teleconferences periodically to inform them about the latest project achievements. We recommend as well sending regular emails to the sponsors providing a brief overview over the project progress.

User integration

- Understanding the target group (needs, wishes, predispositions): In a project that aims to develop a product or service for an end user it is absolutely vital to analyze and understand the target group. Often, the target group is complex in set-up and may have to be subdivided. It is also very important for innovators to keep in mind that the needs and interests of members of the target group may be very different from their own.
- Building long term relationships within a project: In order to improve the success of a project, it is very important to include end users during several stages of the project and keep them involved until the end of it. As a result, the end users will become engaged in the project and may even directly support the market introduction.
- Installing an informal exchange (e.g. regulars' table): Much more than formal ways of user integration, informal approaches will provide authentic insights.
- Employing users as development partners: Making the user a development partner is all but easy. However, if successful, it is the most effective and efficient way of user integration.

Product focus

- A good mix between innovation level and market compatibility: In most innovation projects, both aspects are very important. On the one hand, one should realize something new and innovative that solves a problem and meets a need in a new and effective way. On the other hand, this solution should be very well aligned to the current market development. The right mix between breakthrough and incremental innovation thus is the key to success.
- Systemic product development: Innovators are system designers. Thus, rather than just focusing on particular product features they must have the complete system solution in mind, including product purchase, learning, maintenance and social and technical interfaces.
- Adaptation to the living environment and the habits of the target group: In order to keep the product focused, it is important to consider the physical, social and emotional environment of the target group, and at best test and evaluate the final prototype in a real environment. This ensures a continuous market plausibility reflection of the state of the art of the innovation, and a consideration of fixed market parameters as early as possible.

Market introduction

- Naming one responsible promoter: In the set-up of the project, it is advisable to name one person as responsible for the go-to-market phase, who will lead the action to bring the final project prototype into the market.
- Finding and contacting allied partners as early as possible: Despite having all the members of the value chain represented in the consortium, it is vital to look for as many allies as possible as the market introduction is complex, resource consuming and core to the product and project success. This will help to hit the market needs and meet all stakeholder demands, but also support fast and resource-efficient market introduction.

Reference

Moritz, E.F.: Holistische Innovation. Konzept, Methodik und Beispiele. Springer, Heidelberg (2009)

About the Editor

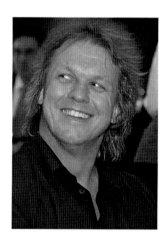

Prof. Dr. Eckehard Fozzy Moritz has studied Mechanical Engineering at the Technical University of Munich, and received his Doctorate Degree at the Tokyo Institute of Technology. He is currently director of Innovationsmanufaktur GmbH, a company masterminding, moderating, and facilitating innovation projects for public sponsors and foundations, for companies like BMW, Bosch and BASF, and for government agencies in Germany, Italy, Spain and Mexico. He holds a honorary professorship from Qufu University, China, and is adjunct professor at the Universidad de las Américas, Puebla, Mexico. Prof. Moritz has been chairman of the 6th World Conference of the International Sports Engineering Association, and has been teaching and consulting at universities in 27 countries world-wide. He is author of the book "Holistische Innovation", Springer-Verlag 2009, in which a new methodology to deal with complex innovation challenges is introduced.

E. F. Moritz (ed.), *Assistive Technologies for the Interaction of the Elderly*, Advanced Technologies and Societal Change, DOI: 10.1007/978-3-319-00678-9, © Springer International Publishing Switzerland 2014

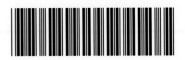